GUT HEALTH
COOKBOOK FOR WOMEN

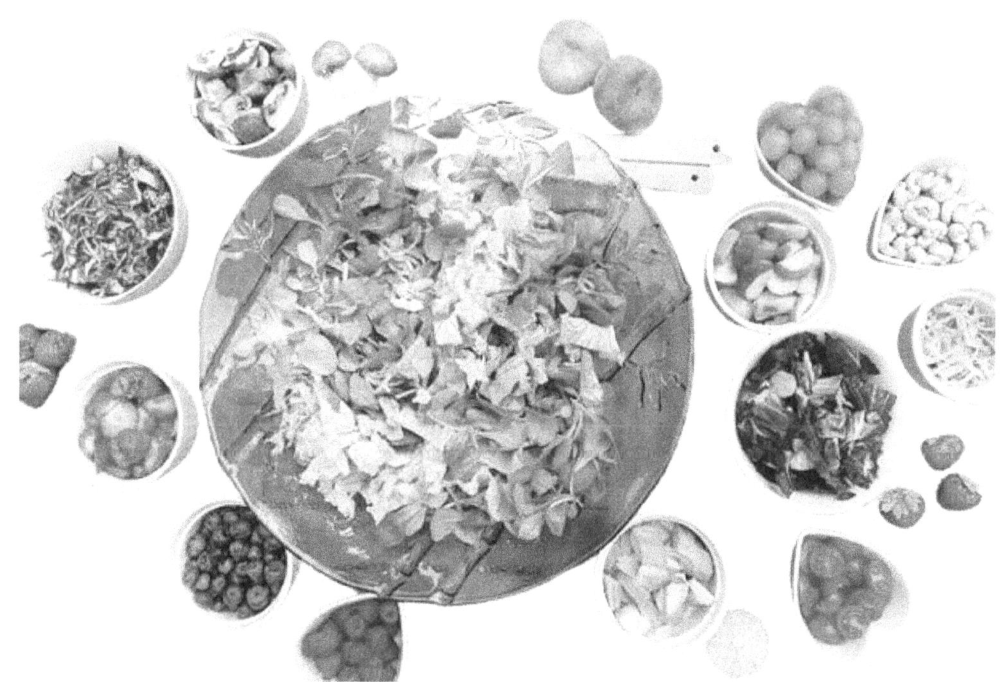

DR. VICKIE STOCK

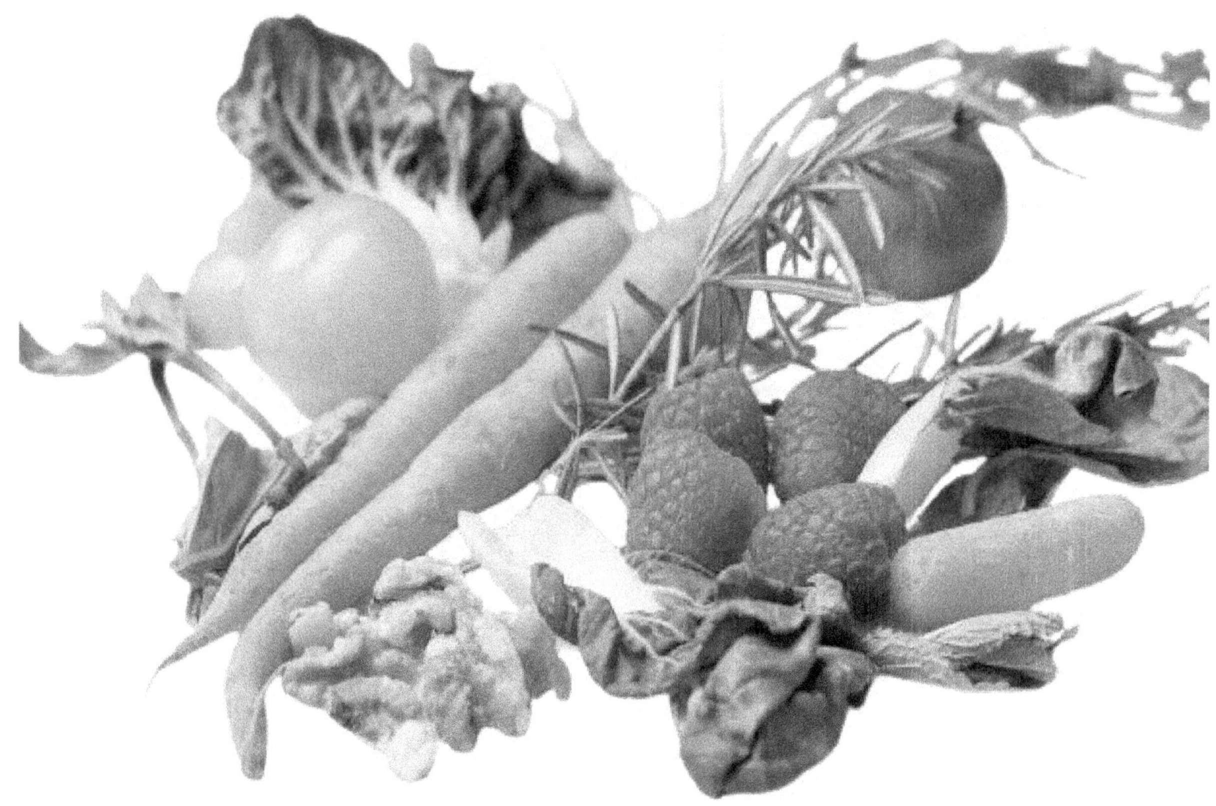

TABLE OF CONTENT

CHAPTER ONE: Understanding Gut Health

Introduction to Gut Health

Gut health has emerged as a cornerstone of overall well-being, with a growing body of research highlighting its pivotal role in maintaining a healthy and balanced life. The gastrointestinal system, often referred to as the gut, is a complex network of organs, tissues, and trillions of microorganisms collectively known as the microbiome. This intricate ecosystem plays a crucial role not only in digestion but also in influencing various aspects of our health, including immune function, mental well-being, and hormonal balance.

The significance of gut health, especially for women, cannot be overstated. Women's bodies undergo unique physiological changes, such as menstruation, pregnancy, and menopause, which can profoundly impact the gut. The intricate interplay between the gut and hormonal fluctuations underscores the need for tailored approaches to support women's digestive health.

The microbiome, a diverse community of bacteria, viruses, fungi, and other microorganisms residing in the gut, has gained attention for its profound impact on health. These microorganisms contribute to digestion, nutrient absorption, and the synthesis of essential vitamins. Moreover, they play a pivotal role in maintaining a robust immune system, protecting against pathogens, and even influencing mood and cognitive function through the gut-brain axis.

Understanding gut health involves recognizing the delicate balance within this microbial community. Disruptions to this equilibrium, often caused by factors like poor dietary choices, stress, antibiotics, and environmental influences, can lead to an imbalance in the microbiome—a condition known as dysbiosis. Dysbiosis has been linked to various health issues, including digestive disorders, autoimmune diseases, and mental health disorders.

Common gut health issues that affect women, such as Irritable Bowel Syndrome (IBS), Leaky Gut Syndrome, and Candida overgrowth, underscore the need for proactive measures to support digestive wellness. The relationship between gut health and hormonal balance is particularly noteworthy, as imbalances in estrogen and progesterone can influence gut function and vice versa.

Assessing one's gut health involves paying attention to subtle signs and symptoms, ranging from digestive discomfort and irregular bowel movements to skin issues and fatigue. Diagnostic tests, including stool analysis and microbiome testing, provide valuable insights into the composition and health of the gut microbiota.

As we delve into the chapters of this cookbook, it is essential to recognize that achieving optimal gut health is a holistic journey. From mindful food choices and cooking techniques to lifestyle modifications that mitigate stress, every aspect plays a role in fostering a thriving gut ecosystem. The recipes and guidelines presented herein are crafted to empower women in cultivating a gut-friendly lifestyle, embracing the symbiotic relationship between nutrition, wellness, and digestive health.

The Importance of Gut Health for Women

Gut health stands at the forefront of overall well-being, and for women, understanding and nurturing the intricate ecosystem within the digestive system is paramount. The gastrointestinal tract, often referred to as the gut, is not merely a system responsible for processing and absorbing nutrients; it serves as a dynamic hub influencing various aspects of a woman's health throughout her life.

One of the key areas where gut health plays a critical role for women is in hormonal balance. Women undergo unique hormonal fluctuations during different life stages, such as menstruation, pregnancy, and menopause. The gut microbiome, a vast community of microorganisms residing in the digestive tract, has been shown to interact with and influence hormonal regulation.

A well-balanced microbiome contributes to the proper metabolism of hormones like estrogen and progesterone, fostering hormonal harmony. Conversely, an imbalanced gut can contribute to hormonal disruptions, potentially exacerbating conditions such as PMS, irregular menstrual cycles, and menopausal symptoms.

The impact of gut health on reproductive health is profound. Research suggests that a healthy and diverse gut microbiome may positively influence fertility and pregnancy outcomes. Maintaining an optimal balance of beneficial bacteria in the gut can enhance nutrient absorption, support a healthy immune system, and create an environment conducive to reproductive health.

Beyond hormonal and reproductive considerations, the gut plays a pivotal role in immune function. A substantial portion of the body's immune cells resides in the gut-associated lymphoid tissue (GALT), and the microbiome plays a crucial role in training and modulating the immune system. For women, a robust immune system is essential for defending against infections, supporting a healthy pregnancy, and overall resilience to illnesses.

Moreover, gut health has implications for mental well-being, an area of particular significance for women who are more prone to conditions like anxiety and depression. The gut-brain axis, a bidirectional communication system between the gut and the brain, highlights the profound impact of gut health on mood and cognitive function. A balanced and diverse microbiome is associated with better mental health outcomes, emphasizing the need for women to prioritize their gut health for overall emotional well-being.

Gut-Brain Connection

The gut-brain connection represents a fascinating and intricate communication network that underscores the interdependence of the digestive system and the central nervous system. This bidirectional communication highway, linking the gut and the brain, has far-reaching implications for various aspects of human health, including mental well-being, cognitive function, and emotional balance.

At the core of the gut-brain connection is the enteric nervous system (ENS), often referred to as the "second brain." The ENS, an extensive network of neurons lining the gastrointestinal tract, operates independently but is in constant communication with the central nervous system through the vagus nerve. This intricate web of communication allows the gut to influence the brain and vice versa, shaping both physical and mental health.

One of the key players in the gut-brain axis is the gut microbiome, a diverse community of trillions of microorganisms residing in the digestive tract. These microbes play a crucial role in producing neurotransmitters, the chemical messengers that regulate mood, cognition, and stress response. For instance, the gut microbiota produces serotonin, often referred to as the "feel-good" neurotransmitter, influencing mood and emotional well-being. Imbalances in the gut microbiome have been associated with conditions such as anxiety, depression, and stress-related disorders, highlighting the significance of maintaining a healthy gut for optimal mental health.

Moreover, the gut-brain connection plays a role in the body's stress response. Chronic stress can impact the balance of the gut microbiome, leading to dysbiosis, which, in turn, may contribute to stress-related disorders. Techniques such as mindfulness and relaxation, which positively influence the gut-brain axis, have been shown to support a healthier gut microbiome and mitigate the effects of chronic stress.

Dietary choices also play a crucial role in shaping the gut-brain connection. Certain foods, such as those rich in fiber and prebiotics, support the growth of beneficial gut bacteria, fostering a healthy microbiome. On the other hand, diets high in processed foods and sugars have been associated with negative effects on gut health and mental well-being.

Understanding the gut-brain connection opens up new avenues for promoting mental health through lifestyle and dietary interventions. As women navigate the challenges of daily life, recognizing the profound impact of their gut health on their mental well-being becomes crucial. This cookbook provides a toolkit for women to nourish their gut and, in turn, support a healthy and resilient mind, fostering a harmonious balance between the gut and the brain.

Section 2

What is the Microbiome?

The microbiome, a term that has gained prominence in the realm of health and wellness, refers to the vast and diverse community of microorganisms that inhabit various parts of the human body. However, when we speak of "the microbiome," we often specifically refer to the complex ecosystem residing in the digestive tract, known as the gut microbiome. This intricate assembly of bacteria, viruses, fungi, and other microorganisms collaborates in a symbiotic relationship with the human body, influencing health and functioning as a dynamic biological entity.

Trillions of microorganisms call the human gut home, collectively forming a thriving community that plays a pivotal role in digestion, nutrient absorption, and overall immune function. The gut microbiome is a dynamic and ever-changing ecosystem influenced by factors such as diet, lifestyle, genetics, and environmental exposures. It adapts to various stimuli, constantly shaping its composition and diversity.

The microbiome contributes significantly to the breakdown of complex carbohydrates and fibers that our bodies cannot digest on their own. This process results in the production of short-chain fatty acids (SCFAs), essential compounds that support the health of the gut lining and provide a source of energy for the body. Additionally, the microbiome synthesizes certain vitamins, such as B vitamins and vitamin K, contributing to the overall nutritional status of the host.

Beyond its role in digestion and nutrient metabolism, the gut microbiome is intricately connected to other aspects of health, including immune function. A balanced and diverse microbiome helps educate and regulate the immune system, promoting a robust defense against pathogens while preventing inappropriate responses to harmless substances. Disruptions in the microbiome's balance, known as dysbiosis, have been linked to various health issues, including inflammatory bowel diseases, allergies, and autoimmune conditions.

The importance of the gut microbiome extends beyond physical health to mental well-being. Research has unveiled the profound connection between the gut and the brain, known as the gut-brain axis, where the microbiome influences neurotransmitter production and plays a role in regulating mood and cognitive function. An imbalance in the microbiome has been associated with conditions such as anxiety, depression, and stress-related disorders.

Understanding the microbiome unveils a new frontier in healthcare, emphasizing the significance of maintaining a balanced and diverse community of microorganisms for overall well-being. This cookbook aims to empower women with insights and recipes that not only support digestive health but also contribute to the flourishing of the microbiome, fostering a harmonious relationship between the human body and its microscopic inhabitants.

Role of Microbes in Gut Health

The gut, often referred to as the second brain, is a complex ecosystem where trillions of microorganisms, collectively known as the gut microbiota, form a thriving community that profoundly influences human health. The role of microbes in gut health is multifaceted, extending beyond mere digestion to impact various physiological functions and overall well-being.

Digestion and Nutrient Absorption:

At the forefront of the microbiome's role is its contribution to the digestive process. Certain microbes aid in breaking down complex carbohydrates, fibers, and other indigestible components of the diet that the human body, on its own, cannot metabolize. This microbial digestion results in the production of short-chain fatty acids (SCFAs), which not only serve as an energy source for the host but also contribute to the health of the gut lining.

Immune System Modulation:

The gut microbiota plays a crucial role in training and modulating the immune system. A harmonious relationship between the host and the microbiome is essential for maintaining a robust defense against pathogens while preventing inappropriate immune responses to harmless substances. Microbes in the gut stimulate the development and maturation of immune cells, contributing to the overall resilience of the immune system.

Synthesis of Bioactive Compounds:

Microbes within the gut are capable of synthesizing various bioactive compounds, including certain vitamins and neurotransmitters. For instance, the microbiome contributes to the production of B vitamins and vitamin K, essential for various physiological functions. Moreover, specific strains of bacteria in the gut are involved in the synthesis of neurotransmitters such as serotonin, impacting mood, stress response, and overall mental well-being.

Barrier Function and Protection:

The gut microbiota plays a crucial role in maintaining the integrity of the gut barrier. A healthy microbiome helps prevent the infiltration of harmful pathogens and toxins into the bloodstream, contributing to overall gut health. Dysbiosis, or an imbalance in the microbial community, can compromise the gut barrier function, potentially leading to inflammation and various digestive issues.

Metabolism and Weight Regulation:

Emerging research suggests a connection between the composition of the gut microbiota and metabolism. Certain microbes may influence how the body stores and utilizes energy, impacting weight regulation. An imbalance in the microbiome has been associated with conditions such as obesity and metabolic disorders. Understanding the intricate role of microbes in gut health emphasizes the need to nurture and support a diverse and balanced microbiome.

This cookbook is crafted to provide women with recipes and dietary strategies that not only promote digestive wellness but also contribute to fostering a thriving microbial community within the gut, paving the way for holistic health and vitality.

Irritable Bowel Syndrome (IBS) is a prevalent and multifaceted gastrointestinal disorder that affects a significant number of individuals, with women being more commonly affected than men. This condition is characterized by a constellation of symptoms that can range from abdominal pain and bloating to changes in bowel habits, making it a challenging and often misunderstood aspect of digestive health.

Symptoms and Diagnosis:

The symptoms of IBS can vary widely from person to person, making it a complex condition to diagnose. Common symptoms include abdominal pain or discomfort, bloating, and alterations in bowel habits such as diarrhea, constipation, or a combination of both. The Rome Criteria, a set of guidelines for diagnosing functional gastrointestinal disorders, is often utilized to identify IBS based on specific symptom patterns.

Hormonal Influence:

Women, in particular, are more susceptible to IBS, and hormonal factors play a significant role in the manifestation of symptoms. Changes in estrogen levels, which occur during menstruation, pregnancy, and menopause, can impact the sensitivity of the gut and contribute to symptom exacerbation. The hormonal influence underscores the need for personalized approaches in managing IBS in women.

Gut-Brain Axis and Stress:

The gut-brain axis, a bidirectional communication system between the gut and the central nervous system, plays a crucial role in IBS. Stress and emotional factors can trigger or exacerbate symptoms, highlighting the intricate connection between the mind and the gut.

Managing stress through relaxation techniques, mindfulness, and lifestyle adjustments is a key component of IBS management.

Dietary Triggers:

Certain foods and dietary patterns can act as triggers for IBS symptoms. Common culprits include high-fat foods, spicy foods, dairy products, and artificial sweeteners. Identifying and avoiding individual dietary triggers can be instrumental in symptom management. Additionally, adopting a low-FODMAP (fermentable oligosaccharides, disaccharides, monosaccharides, and polyols) diet has shown effectiveness in reducing symptoms for many individuals with IBS.

Lifestyle Modifications:

Lifestyle factors play a crucial role in managing IBS. Regular physical activity, maintaining a consistent sleep schedule, and staying hydrated contribute to overall well-being and can positively impact digestive health. Establishing a routine and recognizing patterns in symptom occurrence can aid individuals in managing and mitigating the impact of IBS on their daily lives.

Medical Approaches:

While there is no cure for IBS, various medical approaches can help alleviate symptoms. Medications such as antispasmodics, laxatives, and certain antidepressants may be prescribed based on the predominant symptoms. Probiotics, which promote a healthy balance of gut bacteria, have also shown promise in managing IBS symptoms.

Leaky Gut Syndrome

Leaky Gut Syndrome, a term that has gained attention in the realm of digestive health, refers to increased intestinal permeability, where the lining of the intestines becomes more porous than usual. This condition allows substances such as bacteria, toxins, and undigested food particles to pass through the intestinal wall and enter the bloodstream.

While not universally recognized as a formal medical diagnosis, the concept of Leaky Gut Syndrome underscores the potential connections between gut health and systemic well-being.

Intestinal Barrier Dysfunction:

The intestines have a crucial role in nutrient absorption while serving as a protective barrier against harmful substances. The lining of the intestines is comprised of tightly packed cells held together by junctions. In Leaky Gut Syndrome, these junctions become loose, allowing substances to permeate the intestinal wall. This breach in the barrier can lead to inflammation and trigger various health issues.

Causes and Contributing Factors:

Leaky Gut Syndrome is thought to result from a combination of genetic, environmental, and lifestyle factors. Chronic stress, poor diet, excessive alcohol consumption, and the use of certain medications, particularly nonsteroidal anti-inflammatory drugs (NSAIDs) and antibiotics, are among the factors implicated in the development of intestinal permeability. Additionally, conditions such as celiac disease, Crohn's disease, and irritable bowel syndrome (IBS) may contribute to Leaky Gut Syndrome.

Systemic Impact:

The permeability of the intestinal barrier allows substances to enter the bloodstream that would typically be restricted. This can trigger an immune response, leading to inflammation throughout the body. The systemic impact of Leaky Gut Syndrome is believed to contribute to a range of health issues, including autoimmune conditions, allergies, skin disorders, and even neurological symptoms. The connections between the gut and other organ systems highlight the potential far-reaching consequences of compromised gut health.

Symptoms and Recognition:

Recognizing Leaky Gut Syndrome can be challenging, as symptoms can be diverse and nonspecific. Common signs include digestive issues such as bloating, gas, and abdominal pain, as well as systemic symptoms like fatigue, joint pain, and skin problems. Given the broad spectrum of symptoms, healthcare providers may explore various diagnostic approaches, including assessing symptoms, conducting laboratory tests, and sometimes employing intestinal permeability tests.

Management and Treatment:

While there is ongoing research into Leaky Gut Syndrome, the management typically involves addressing underlying causes and supporting gut health. Dietary modifications, such as adopting a low-inflammatory diet and incorporating gut-healing foods, can be beneficial. Probiotics, which promote a healthy balance of gut bacteria, may also play a role in restoring intestinal health. Lifestyle changes, including stress management and reducing exposure to potential triggers, are essential components of a holistic approach to managing Leaky Gut Syndrome.

Candida Overgrowth

Candida overgrowth, caused by an excessive proliferation of Candida, a type of yeast, in the digestive tract, is a condition that has garnered attention in the realm of gut health. Candida is a natural component of the gut microbiome, but an imbalance in its population can lead to overgrowth, potentially giving rise to a range of symptoms and health issues.

Candida in the Gut Microbiome:

Candida is a yeast that normally resides in the gut alongside other microorganisms. In a balanced microbiome, Candida coexists harmoniously with bacteria and other fungi. However, various factors, such as a weakened immune system, prolonged use of antibiotics, hormonal changes, and high sugar diets, can disrupt this balance, allowing Candida to proliferate.

Common Causes and Risk Factors:

Several factors contribute to Candida overgrowth. The use of broad-spectrum antibiotics, which can deplete beneficial bacteria in the gut, creates an environment conducive to Candida proliferation. Hormonal fluctuations, as seen in women during pregnancy, menstruation, or the use of birth control pills, may also increase susceptibility. Diets high in refined sugars and carbohydrates provide an ample food source for Candida, promoting its growth.

Symptoms of Candida Overgrowth:

Candida overgrowth can manifest in a variety of symptoms, making it challenging to diagnose. Common symptoms include recurrent yeast infections, digestive issues such as bloating and gas, fatigue, brain fog, and skin conditions. These symptoms can be nonspecific, often leading to difficulty in pinpointing Candida overgrowth as the root cause.

Diagnostic Challenges:

Diagnosing Candida overgrowth can be challenging due to the lack of definitive tests. Healthcare providers often rely on a combination of symptoms, medical history, and sometimes specific diagnostic tests, such as stool or blood tests, to assess the presence of Candida overgrowth. However, it's important to note that the diagnostic process may vary, and healthcare providers approach it based on individual cases.

Treatment and Management:

Managing Candida overgrowth typically involves a multifaceted approach. Dietary changes are often central to the strategy, including reducing the intake of sugars, refined carbohydrates, and yeasted foods. Probiotics, which introduce beneficial bacteria to the gut, may help restore microbial balance. Antifungal medications may be prescribed in severe cases, especially if the overgrowth has led to systemic issues.

Preventive Measures:

Adopting lifestyle and dietary habits that promote a healthy gut microbiome is key to preventing Candida overgrowth. This includes maintaining a balanced diet rich in fiber, managing stress, avoiding unnecessary antibiotic use, and supporting the immune system through regular exercise and adequate sleep.

This cookbook endeavors to empower individuals, particularly women who may be more susceptible to hormonal influences, with recipes and dietary guidance that align with principles supportive of gut health. By offering a collection of delicious and nutritious recipes, the cookbook aims to contribute to a gut-friendly lifestyle that fosters balance, resilience, and optimal microbial harmony within the digestive tract.

Section 4

Factors Affecting Gut Health

Diet and Nutrition

The adage "you are what you eat" holds profound truth when it comes to the intricate relationship between diet, nutrition, and overall health.

Diet plays a pivotal role in shaping the composition and function of the gut microbiome, influencing not only digestive health but also various aspects of physical and mental well-being.

Impact on the Gut Microbiome:

The gut microbiome, a complex community of trillions of microorganisms residing in the digestive tract, is profoundly influenced by dietary choices. A diet rich in fiber from fruits, vegetables, and whole grains provides essential nutrients that support the growth of beneficial bacteria. These microbes, in turn, contribute to digestion, nutrient absorption, and the synthesis of bioactive compounds crucial for overall health.

Probiotics and Fermented Foods:

Probiotics, beneficial bacteria that confer health benefits, are commonly found in fermented foods like yogurt, kefir, sauerkraut, and kimchi. Including these foods in the diet introduces live cultures that can positively impact the gut microbiota. Probiotics contribute to microbial diversity, enhance the balance of the microbiome, and may offer protection against harmful pathogens.

Prebiotics and Fiber-Rich Foods:

Prebiotics are non-digestible fibers that serve as fuel for beneficial bacteria in the gut. Foods high in prebiotics include garlic, onions, leeks, bananas, and asparagus. Incorporating these fiber-rich foods into the diet promotes the growth of specific microbes that contribute to gut health. The synergistic relationship between prebiotics and probiotics is crucial for maintaining microbial balance.

Balancing Macronutrients:

The balance of macronutrients—carbohydrates, proteins, and fats—plays a role in supporting gut health.

A diet excessively high in saturated fats and low in fiber can negatively impact the microbiome, promoting the growth of less beneficial bacteria. Striking a balance between healthy fats, lean proteins, and complex carbohydrates contributes to overall nutritional harmony.

Hydration and Gut Function:

Adequate hydration is fundamental for digestive health. Water facilitates the movement of food through the digestive tract, helps in nutrient absorption, and supports the overall function of the gastrointestinal system. Staying hydrated is essential for maintaining optimal gut function and preventing issues such as constipation.

Nutrient-Dense Whole Foods:

Choosing nutrient-dense whole foods over processed and refined options is a key principle of a gut-friendly diet. Whole foods, such as fruits, vegetables, lean proteins, and whole grains, provide a rich array of vitamins, minerals, antioxidants, and other bioactive compounds that contribute to overall health and support the gut microbiome.

Individualized Approaches:

Recognizing the individual variability in dietary needs is essential. While general principles guide a gut-healthy diet, individuals may respond differently to specific foods. Tailoring dietary choices to accommodate individual preferences, tolerances, and sensitivities ensures a sustainable and personalized approach to nutrition.

Diet and nutrition serve as the bedrock of gut health and overall well-being. This cookbook endeavors to provide a repertoire of recipes aligned with principles that support digestive resilience, promoting a holistic and individualized approach to nutrition for optimal health.

Lifestyle and Stress

between lifestyle and stress there is a pivotal role in shaping not only our mental and emotional well-being but also the health of our gut. Lifestyle choices, including habits related to diet, physical activity, sleep, and stress management, collectively contribute to the delicate balance within the gut microbiome and influence overall digestive health.

Stress and the Gut-Brain Axis:

The gut-brain axis, a complex bidirectional communication system between the gut and the central nervous system, underscores the profound impact of stress on digestive health. Chronic stress can trigger physiological responses that affect gut motility, increase gut permeability, and alter the composition of the gut microbiota. These changes may contribute to conditions such as irritable bowel syndrome (IBS), emphasizing the need for effective stress management strategies.

Mindful Eating and Digestive Harmony:

The practice of mindful eating is a valuable aspect of a gut-friendly lifestyle. Eating slowly, savoring each bite, and being attuned to hunger and fullness cues can positively influence the digestive process. Additionally, mindful eating fosters a relaxed state, reducing the likelihood of stress-related disruptions to digestion.

Regular Physical Activity and Gut Health:

Regular exercise is not only beneficial for cardiovascular health and weight management but also plays a role in supporting gut health. Physical activity has been associated with a more diverse and balanced gut microbiome. The mechanisms linking exercise and gut health include improved gut motility, enhanced microbial diversity, and a potential reduction in inflammation.

Sleep Quality and Circadian Rhythms:

Adequate and quality sleep is essential for overall well-being, including digestive health. Disruptions to circadian rhythms and irregular sleep patterns can impact the gut microbiome and contribute to conditions like dysbiosis. Establishing a consistent sleep schedule and prioritizing sufficient sleep duration are crucial components of a lifestyle that supports gut health.

Stress Management Techniques:

Effective stress management is paramount for maintaining gut health. Techniques such as meditation, deep breathing exercises, yoga, and other relaxation practices can mitigate the physiological effects of stress on the gastrointestinal system. These approaches promote a state of calm and contribute to a more favorable environment within the gut.

Social Connections and Emotional Well-Being:

Social connections and emotional well-being are integral aspects of a holistic lifestyle that supports gut health. Positive social interactions and emotional resilience contribute to a balanced nervous system, fostering an environment conducive to optimal digestion. Cultivating meaningful relationships and engaging in activities that bring joy contribute to overall emotional well-being.

Hydration and Gut Function:

Proper hydration is a lifestyle habit that supports gut function. Water is essential for maintaining mucosal integrity, promoting the movement of food through the digestive tract, and aiding in nutrient absorption. Staying hydrated contributes to optimal gut health and is a simple yet impactful aspect of a gut-friendly lifestyle.

Hormonal Changes

Hormonal changes are a natural and inevitable part of a woman's life, influencing various physiological processes, including digestive health. Understanding how hormonal fluctuations, occurring during menstruation, pregnancy, and menopause, impact the digestive system is crucial for tailoring lifestyle and dietary choices to support women's overall well-being.

Menstrual Cycle and Digestive Symptoms:

The menstrual cycle involves intricate hormonal shifts, primarily those of estrogen and progesterone. Many women experience changes in digestive patterns throughout the menstrual cycle. Some may notice bloating, changes in bowel habits, or abdominal discomfort during the premenstrual phase. These symptoms are often linked to hormonal variations affecting gut motility and water balance.

Pregnancy and Digestive Adaptations:

Pregnancy is characterized by significant hormonal changes to support fetal development. The surge in hormones, including human chorionic gonadotropin (hCG), progesterone, and estrogen, can impact the digestive system. Women may experience symptoms such as nausea, heartburn, and constipation. Progesterone, in particular, relaxes smooth muscles, slowing down the digestive process and contributing to constipation.

Postpartum Hormonal Adjustments:

After childbirth, hormonal fluctuations continue as the body transitions to a non-pregnant state. While some digestive issues experienced during pregnancy may resolve, postpartum hormonal changes, including fluctuations in estrogen and prolactin, can influence bowel habits and digestion. Supportive dietary choices are essential during this phase of recovery.

Menopause and Gastrointestinal Changes:

Menopause, marked by the cessation of menstruation, brings about a significant decline in estrogen levels. This hormonal shift can influence various aspects of women's health, including changes in the gastrointestinal tract. Some women may experience symptoms such as bloating, indigestion, and altered bowel habits during menopause. Hormonal replacement therapy and lifestyle modifications can be considered to manage these changes.

Estrogen and Gut Microbiome:

Estrogen, a key female sex hormone, plays a role in shaping the gut microbiome. Research suggests that fluctuations in estrogen levels can influence the composition of gut bacteria. A balanced and diverse gut microbiome is essential for digestive health, nutrient absorption, and immune function. Supporting the microbiome through dietary choices becomes crucial during hormonal changes.

Impact of Hormonal Contraceptives:

Hormonal contraceptives, such as birth control pills, influence hormonal levels to prevent pregnancy. These contraceptives may impact the gut microbiome and digestive function. Women using hormonal contraceptives may experience changes in appetite, nutrient absorption, and gut motility. Individual responses vary, and consideration of gut health is relevant when choosing contraceptive methods.

Nutritional Support During Hormonal Changes:

Proper nutrition is a cornerstone for supporting women's digestive health during hormonal changes. Including fiber-rich foods, staying hydrated, and consuming a variety of nutrients are foundational principles. Addressing specific symptoms, such as bloating or constipation, may involve dietary modifications tailored to individual needs.

Section 5

Assessing Your Gut Health

Evaluating and understanding your gut health involves considering a myriad of factors that collectively contribute to the balance and functionality of your digestive system. While there is no one-size-fits-all approach, assessing your gut health encompasses various aspects, allowing for a holistic exploration of well-being.

Digestive Symptoms:

Start by paying attention to your digestive symptoms. Common indicators of potential gut issues include bloating, gas, abdominal discomfort, irregular bowel habits, and changes in stool consistency. The presence and frequency of these symptoms can offer insights into the overall health of your digestive system.

Dietary Habits:

Your dietary choices play a pivotal role in shaping gut health. Evaluate the composition of your diet, considering the intake of fiber, fruits, vegetables, and fermented foods. A diet rich in these elements supports the growth of beneficial bacteria in the gut, contributing to a diverse and balanced microbiome.

Hydration:

Adequate hydration is essential for digestive health. Water facilitates the movement of food through the digestive tract, supports the absorption of nutrients, and helps maintain the mucosal integrity of the intestines. Assess your daily water intake and ensure it aligns with your body's hydration needs.

Stress Levels:

Chronic stress can adversely affect gut health through the gut-brain axis. Assess your stress levels and identify stressors in your life. Incorporating stress management techniques, such as mindfulness, meditation, or regular physical activity, can positively impact the balance within the gut.

Sleep Patterns:

Quality sleep is integral to overall well-being, including gut health. Evaluate your sleep patterns, considering both duration and quality. Establishing a consistent sleep routine and prioritizing sufficient sleep can contribute to optimal digestive function.

Physical Activity:

Regular physical activity has been linked to a more diverse and balanced gut microbiome. Assess your level of physical activity and consider incorporating regular exercise into your routine. This not only benefits your gut but also supports overall health.

Medication History:

Review your medication history, including the use of antibiotics, nonsteroidal anti-inflammatory drugs (NSAIDs), and other medications. Certain medications can impact the balance of the gut microbiota. If you have a history of frequent antibiotic use, consider strategies to support gut health, such as probiotic supplementation and dietary adjustments.

Symptoms Beyond the Gut:

Acknowledge symptoms beyond the gut that may be indicative of systemic issues related to gut health.

Skin conditions, autoimmune disorders, and even mood disorders can be influenced by the health of your gut. Assessing these broader symptoms provides a more comprehensive picture of your overall well-being.

Consultation with Healthcare Providers:

If you have persistent or concerning symptoms, consider consulting with healthcare providers specializing in gut health, such as gastroenterologists or registered dietitians. Diagnostic tests, including stool analyses and imaging studies, may be recommended to assess specific aspects of your digestive health.

Genetic and Family History:

Consider your genetic and family history, as certain conditions related to gut health may have a hereditary component. Understanding your predispositions can inform preventive measures and tailored approaches to support your gut health.

Symptoms of Poor Gut Health

The gut, often regarded as the body's second brain, plays a pivotal role in overall well-being.

Symptoms of poor gut health can manifest in various ways, extending beyond digestive discomfort to impact diverse aspects of physical and even mental health. Recognizing these symptoms is essential for addressing underlying issues and fostering optimal gut function.

Digestive Discomfort:

Unpleasant digestive symptoms are key indicators of poor gut health. Bloating, gas, abdominal pain, and cramping are common manifestations. These symptoms may suggest imbalances in the gut microbiome, compromised gut barrier function, or disruptions in the digestive process.

Irregular Bowel Habits:

Changes in bowel habits can signal underlying gut issues. Diarrhea, constipation, or alternating between the two may indicate disruptions in gut motility, inflammation, or imbalances in the gut microbiota. Consistency in bowel habits is a hallmark of a healthy digestive system.

Food Intolerances:

Developing sensitivities or intolerances to certain foods is a potential symptom of poor gut health. Conditions like leaky gut or dysbiosis can lead to heightened immune responses to specific dietary components, resulting in symptoms such as nausea, bloating, or diarrhea after consuming certain foods.

Fatigue and Low Energy:

The gut is intricately connected to energy metabolism, and poor gut health can contribute to feelings of fatigue and low energy. Malabsorption of nutrients, disrupted sleep patterns due to digestive discomfort, or systemic inflammation may all play a role in draining energy levels.

Skin Issues:

Skin conditions like acne, eczema, or psoriasis may be linked to poor gut health. The gut-skin axis highlights the connection between gut imbalances, inflammation, and skin health. Addressing underlying gut issues may contribute to improvements in skin conditions.

Mood Disorders:

The gut-brain axis, a bidirectional communication system between the gut and the brain, influences mental health.

Poor gut health has been associated with mood disorders such as anxiety and depression. Imbalances in the gut microbiota can impact the production of neurotransmitters, affecting mood regulation.

Autoimmune Conditions:

Chronic inflammation stemming from poor gut health can contribute to autoimmune conditions. Conditions like rheumatoid arthritis, inflammatory bowel disease (IBD), and Hashimoto's thyroiditis have been linked to imbalances in the gut microbiome and increased gut permeability.

Nutritional Deficiencies:

Malabsorption and compromised nutrient assimilation are common consequences of poor gut health. Deficiencies in essential nutrients such as vitamins and minerals may manifest as a range of symptoms, including weakness, dizziness, and difficulty concentrating.

Weight Changes:

Unexplained weight loss or gain can be linked to poor gut health. Disruptions in the gut microbiome may impact metabolism, energy extraction from food, and appetite regulation, leading to fluctuations in body weight.

Joint Pain and Inflammation:

Chronic joint pain and inflammation may be associated with poor gut health. In conditions like rheumatoid arthritis, the immune system's response to gut dysbiosis can contribute to systemic inflammation affecting joints.

Diagnostic Tests for Gut Health

Understanding the intricacies of gut health often requires more than recognizing symptoms; it involves employing various diagnostic tests to uncover underlying issues and tailor interventions effectively. From assessing the composition of the gut microbiome to identifying potential inflammation or infections, diagnostic tests play a pivotal role in unraveling the complexities of digestive wellness.

Stool Analysis:

Stool analysis is a fundamental diagnostic tool for evaluating gut health. It provides insights into the composition of the microbiome, identifying the presence of beneficial and harmful bacteria, parasites, and other microorganisms. Stool tests can also assess markers of inflammation and digestion, offering a comprehensive overview of digestive function.

Colonoscopy and Endoscopy:

These invasive procedures involve the insertion of a flexible tube with a camera into the colon (colonoscopy) or upper digestive tract (endoscopy). They allow direct visualization of the digestive organs, facilitating the detection of abnormalities, inflammation, polyps, or other structural issues that may contribute to digestive symptoms.

Blood Tests:

Blood tests can provide valuable information about various aspects of gut health. Elevated levels of inflammatory markers, such as C-reactive protein (CRP) or erythrocyte sedimentation rate (ESR), may indicate inflammation in the digestive tract. Blood tests can also assess nutritional status, identifying potential deficiencies related to malabsorption or dietary patterns.

Breath Tests:

Breath tests are utilized to diagnose conditions such as small intestinal bacterial overgrowth (SIBO) and carbohydrate malabsorption. Patients consume a specific substrate, and the subsequent analysis of breath samples measures the gases produced by bacteria during digestion, offering insights into microbial activity and potential malabsorption.

Imaging Studies:

Radiological imaging studies, such as abdominal ultrasound, CT scans, or magnetic resonance imaging (MRI), can be employed to visualize the structure and function of the digestive organs. These tests help identify structural abnormalities, tumors, or obstructions contributing to digestive symptoms.

Food Sensitivity Testing:

Food sensitivity tests aim to identify specific foods that may trigger immune responses or intolerances. While controversial, some tests measure immunoglobulin G (IgG) antibodies to assess reactions to certain foods. It's important to note that the clinical validity of such tests may vary, and interpretation requires careful consideration.

Genetic Testing:

Genetic testing can offer insights into an individual's susceptibility to certain digestive conditions. For example, genetic markers associated with celiac disease or inflammatory bowel disease (IBD) can be identified. Genetic testing may inform preventive measures or guide personalized interventions based on an individual's genetic predispositions.

Biopsy:

Biopsies involve the collection of small tissue samples from the digestive tract during endoscopic procedures. Histological analysis of these samples can provide detailed information about inflammation, cellular changes, or the presence of specific conditions such as celiac disease or inflammatory bowel disease.

Gastrointestinal Motility Tests:

These tests assess the movement and coordination of the muscles in the digestive tract. Manometry measures pressure changes in the esophagus or colon, providing insights into motility disorders such as achalasia or irritable bowel syndrome (IBS).

Hydrogen Breath Tests:

Used primarily for detecting carbohydrate malabsorption and bacterial overgrowth, hydrogen breath tests measure the levels of hydrogen in breath samples after the ingestion of specific substrates. Elevated hydrogen levels can indicate incomplete digestion or fermentation in the gut.

Interpreting diagnostic test results requires expertise, and healthcare providers use a combination of clinical history, symptoms, and test outcomes to formulate a comprehensive understanding of an individual's gut health. These diagnostic tools empower healthcare professionals to tailor interventions, fostering digestive resilience and overall well-being.

CHAPTER TWO: Building Gut Friendly Kitchen

Stocking Gut-Healthy Ingredients

Stocking your kitchen with gut-healthy ingredients is a pivotal step in fostering optimal digestive well-being. The choices you make in your pantry and refrigerator can significantly impact the health of your gut microbiome, influencing everything from nutrient absorption to immune function. Here's a comprehensive guide to help you fill your shelves with the right foods:

Fiber-Rich Foods

Fiber-rich foods play a crucial role in promoting overall health, particularly in supporting digestive well-being. Found in fruits, vegetables, whole grains, legumes, and nuts, dietary fiber offers a multitude of benefits that extend beyond maintaining regular bowel movements. Here's an exploration of the significance and impact of incorporating fiber-rich foods into your diet:

1. Digestive Health:

One of the primary benefits of consuming fiber-rich foods is their positive impact on digestive health. Fiber adds bulk to the stool, which helps prevent constipation and promotes regular bowel movements. Both soluble and insoluble fiber contribute to the overall function of the digestive system, aiding in the smooth passage of food through the gastrointestinal tract.

2. Weight Management:

Fiber plays a crucial role in weight management and satiety. High-fiber foods take longer to chew, slowing down the eating process and giving the body more time to recognize feelings of fullness. Additionally, fiber adds volume to meals without adding a significant number of calories, helping individuals maintain a healthy weight by promoting a sense of satiety while supporting overall dietary balance.

3. Blood Sugar Regulation:

Soluble fiber, found in foods like oats, beans, and fruits, can help regulate blood sugar levels by slowing the absorption of sugar.

This is particularly beneficial for individuals with diabetes or those at risk of developing insulin resistance. Including fiber-rich foods in your diet can contribute to better blood sugar control and overall metabolic health.

4. Cardiovascular Health:

A diet rich in fiber has been linked to improved cardiovascular health. Soluble fiber helps lower cholesterol levels by binding to cholesterol molecules and removing them from the body. This, in turn, reduces the risk of heart disease and stroke. Additionally, the overall anti-inflammatory and antioxidant properties of fiber contribute to a healthier cardiovascular system.

5. Gut Microbiota Support:

Fiber serves as a prebiotic, providing the necessary fuel for beneficial gut bacteria. These microorganisms play a vital role in maintaining a balanced and diverse microbiome, influencing various aspects of health, including immune function and mental well-being. A diet rich in fiber encourages the growth of these beneficial microbes, fostering a symbiotic relationship that contributes to overall gut health.

6. Disease Prevention:

Regular consumption of fiber-rich foods has been associated with a reduced risk of certain diseases, including colorectal cancer. The protective effects of fiber may be attributed to its ability to promote regular bowel movements, reduce inflammation, and support a healthy gut environment.

Incorporating a variety of fiber-rich foods into your daily meals is a practical and delicious way to support overall health. From colorful fruits and vegetables to whole grains and legumes, the diversity of fiber sources allows for creative and satisfying culinary experiences that contribute to a well-balanced and nourishing diet.

Fermented Foods

Fermented foods have earned a well-deserved reputation as nutritional powerhouses, contributing not only to the enhancement of flavor but also to numerous health benefits. The process of fermentation involves the transformation of food by beneficial bacteria, yeast, or molds, leading to the development of probiotics, enzymes, and other bioactive compounds. Here's a closer look at the significance of incorporating fermented foods into your diet:

1. Probiotic Richness:

Fermented foods are teeming with probiotics, which are live microorganisms providing health benefits when consumed in adequate amounts. These friendly bacteria, such as Lactobacillus and Bifidobacterium, support a healthy balance of gut microbiota. Maintaining a diverse and thriving community of beneficial bacteria in the gut is crucial for digestion, nutrient absorption, and immune function.

2. Gut Health Benefits:

Consuming fermented foods contributes to the establishment of a robust gut microbiome. Probiotics introduced through fermented foods can enhance the population of beneficial bacteria in the intestines, helping to maintain a healthy balance and protect against the overgrowth of harmful microbes. Improved gut health is associated with various positive outcomes, including better digestion, reduced inflammation, and even potential benefits for mental well-being.

3. Nutrient Bioavailability:

Fermentation enhances the bioavailability of certain nutrients in food. For example, the fermentation process can break down compounds known as anti-nutrients, making minerals more accessible for absorption. This improved nutrient bioavailability contributes to better overall nutritional status and supports the body in utilizing essential vitamins and minerals.

4. Digestive Enzymes:

Fermented foods contain digestive enzymes that assist in the breakdown of nutrients during digestion. Enzymes like amylase, protease, and lipase help break down carbohydrates, proteins, and fats, respectively. Incorporating these natural enzymes from fermented foods can aid in the digestion process and support the body's ability to extract nutrients from the foods we eat.

5. Immune System Support:

A significant portion of the immune system resides in the gut, and the health of the gut microbiota plays a crucial role in immune function.

Probiotics derived from fermented foods contribute to immune system modulation, helping to regulate and optimize immune responses. This can result in a more robust defense against infections and a reduced risk of immune-related disorders.

6. Diverse Culinary Options:

Fermented foods offer a wide array of flavors and textures, adding depth to culinary experiences. From tangy sauerkraut and kimchi to creamy yogurt and kefir, incorporating fermented foods into your diet introduces a diverse range of taste sensations. This diversity not only satisfies the palate but also encourages a varied and balanced overall diet.

The inclusion of fermented foods in your diet provides a delicious and healthful way to support gut health, nutrient absorption, and overall well-being. Whether enjoyed as a side dish, condiment, or snack, fermented foods contribute to a holistic approach to nutrition, promoting the symbiotic relationship between our bodies and the beneficial microorganisms within.

Prebiotic Foods

Prebiotic foods are a key component of a gut-healthy diet, playing a pivotal role in nurturing the growth and activity of beneficial bacteria in the digestive system. These non-digestible fibers serve as a source of fuel for probiotics, the live microorganisms that confer health benefits. Including prebiotic-rich foods in your diet contributes to a balanced and flourishing gut microbiome, offering a range of benefits for overall health.

1. Nourishing Beneficial Bacteria:

Prebiotics, primarily in the form of soluble fibers, are not digested in the small intestine. Instead, they reach the colon mostly intact, where they serve as a food source for beneficial bacteria such as Bifidobacteria and Lactobacilli. By nourishing these microbes, prebiotics help to maintain a diverse and robust gut microbiota, promoting a healthy balance between beneficial and potentially harmful bacteria.

2. Supporting Colon Health:

The fermentation of prebiotic fibers in the colon produces short-chain fatty acids (SCFAs), such as butyrate, acetate, and propionate. These SCFAs play a crucial role in supporting colon health by providing an energy source for the cells lining the colon, promoting their integrity and function.

Additionally, SCFAs have anti-inflammatory properties, contributing to a healthier gut environment.

3. Enhanced Mineral Absorption:

Prebiotic fibers can enhance the absorption of minerals, particularly calcium and magnesium. By promoting the solubility and availability of these minerals, prebiotics contribute to bone health and overall mineral balance in the body. This is especially important for women, as adequate mineral intake is crucial for maintaining strong and healthy bones.

4. Regulation of Blood Sugar Levels:

Including prebiotic-rich foods in your diet may help regulate blood sugar levels. The fermentation of these fibers in the colon produces substances that influence glucose metabolism, contributing to improved insulin sensitivity. As a result, prebiotics may play a role in reducing the risk of type 2 diabetes and supporting overall metabolic health.

5. Satiety and Weight Management:

Prebiotic-rich foods contribute to feelings of satiety and can be beneficial for weight management. These fibers add bulk to the diet, promoting a sense of fullness and reducing overall calorie intake. By supporting a healthy balance of gut bacteria, prebiotics may also influence the regulation of appetite hormones, contributing to better weight control.

6. Dietary Sources of Prebiotics:

Common dietary sources of prebiotics include garlic, onions, leeks, asparagus, bananas, and Jerusalem artichokes. These foods are easy to incorporate into various recipes, providing a practical and delicious way to support gut health.

Incorporating a variety of prebiotic-rich foods into your daily meals is a proactive approach to fostering a thriving gut microbiome. By prioritizing these fiber-rich sources, you contribute to a balanced and supportive environment for beneficial bacteria, reaping the rewards of improved digestion, enhanced nutrient absorption, and overall well-being.

Cooking techniques play a crucial role in preserving the nutritional value of foods and promoting gut health. The methods employed in preparing meals can impact the digestibility of ingredients and the overall composition of the diet. Here's a closer look at cooking techniques that contribute to gut health:

1. Gentle Cooking Methods:

Opting for gentle cooking methods, such as steaming, poaching, and simmering, helps retain the integrity of nutrients in foods. These methods involve lower temperatures and shorter cooking times compared to more aggressive techniques like frying or grilling. By preserving the nutritional content of foods, gentle cooking methods ensure that the gut receives a higher concentration of vitamins, minerals, and other essential compounds.

2. Fermentation:

While fermentation is often associated with the preparation of specific foods, such as kimchi, sauerkraut, and yogurt, incorporating fermented ingredients into various dishes enhances both flavor and gut health. Fermentation not only introduces beneficial probiotics into the diet but also breaks down certain compounds in food, making nutrients more accessible and improving digestibility. Including fermented components in meals contributes to a diverse and thriving gut microbiome.

3. Incorporating Prebiotics:

Cooking techniques that involve prebiotic-rich foods, such as onions, garlic, and leeks, can enhance the dietary intake of these essential fibers. Lightly sautéing or incorporating these ingredients into stews and soups allows for the release of prebiotic compounds, supporting the growth of beneficial bacteria in the gut. Pairing prebiotics with probiotic-rich foods creates a synergistic effect, fostering a more balanced and resilient microbiota.

4. Avoiding Harmful Cooking Practices:

Certain cooking practices, such as charring and overcooking, can lead to the formation of potentially harmful compounds, including advanced glycation end-products (AGEs). AGEs are formed when proteins or fats react with sugars at high temperatures. Limiting the consumption of heavily charred or overcooked foods is advisable, as these compounds have been associated with inflammation and may have negative effects on gut health.

5. Emphasizing Whole, Unprocessed Foods:

The foundation of a gut-healthy diet lies in the inclusion of whole, unprocessed foods. These foods retain their natural fiber content, vitamins, and minerals. Cooking techniques that focus on preparing meals from scratch, using fresh and minimally processed ingredients, contribute to the overall nutritional quality of the diet. Whole foods provide a spectrum of nutrients that support gut health and overall well-being.

6. Mindful Meal Preparation:

Practicing mindful meal preparation involves taking the time to plan and cook meals with care. It includes selecting a variety of nutrient-dense ingredients, experimenting with different cooking methods, and being attentive to the overall balance of the diet. Mindful cooking supports a diverse and well-rounded nutritional intake, which is beneficial for gut health.

Choosing cooking techniques that prioritize the preservation of nutrients, incorporate beneficial fermented foods, and avoid potentially harmful practices contributes to a gut-friendly diet. By being mindful of the cooking methods used in meal preparation, individuals can enhance the nutritional value of their diets, supporting digestive health and overall well-being.

The Importance of Cooking Methods

The importance of cooking methods extends far beyond the creation of delicious meals; it significantly influences the nutritional quality, safety, and overall health impact of the foods we consume. The choice of cooking techniques can determine the retention of essential nutrients, the formation of potentially harmful compounds, and even the overall digestibility of our meals. Here's a closer exploration of the vital role cooking methods play in our diets:

1. Nutrient Retention:

Different cooking methods have varying effects on the nutrient content of foods. Some nutrients are sensitive to heat, water, or air exposure, and their levels can diminish during cooking. For example, boiling vegetables may cause the loss of water-soluble vitamins like vitamin C.

On the other hand, methods like steaming, microwaving, or grilling at lower temperatures can help preserve the nutritional integrity of foods, ensuring that essential vitamins and minerals remain available for absorption.

2. Impact on Digestibility:

Cooking alters the physical structure of foods, breaking down complex compounds into more digestible forms. Heat softens the texture of fibrous vegetables and starches, making them easier for the digestive system to process. Proper cooking can enhance the availability of nutrients, supporting efficient digestion and nutrient absorption in the gastrointestinal tract.

3. Reduction of Anti-Nutrients:

Certain foods contain anti-nutrients, compounds that can interfere with the absorption of nutrients. Cooking can help neutralize or reduce these anti-nutrients, making the nutrients in the food more bioavailable. For instance, soaking and cooking legumes can decrease levels of compounds like lectins and phytates, which can hinder the absorption of minerals.

4. Food Safety:

Cooking is a crucial step in ensuring food safety by eliminating harmful bacteria, parasites, and viruses present in raw ingredients. Proper cooking temperatures destroy pathogens, reducing the risk of foodborne illnesses. Techniques like roasting, baking, grilling, and sautéing can achieve the necessary temperatures to make food safe for consumption.

5. Flavor Development:

Cooking methods contribute to the development of flavors, textures, and aromas in foods. Techniques such as roasting, searing, and caramelization can enhance the taste and appeal of dishes. The sensory experience of well-cooked food can positively influence eating habits and overall satisfaction, encouraging individuals to maintain a diverse and balanced diet.

6. Culinary Creativity:

Cooking methods provide a palette for culinary creativity, allowing individuals to explore a wide range of flavors and textures. Experimenting with various techniques, from grilling and broiling to braising and steaming, enables the creation of diverse and enjoyable meals.

This variety not only adds excitement to the dining experience but also encourages the consumption of a broad spectrum of nutrients.

The importance of cooking methods lies in their profound impact on the nutritional quality, safety, and enjoyment of the foods we eat. By choosing appropriate cooking techniques, individuals can maximize the benefits of their diets, supporting optimal nutrient intake, digestion, and overall well-being.

Avoiding Harmful Cooking Practices

Avoiding harmful cooking practices is essential for preserving the nutritional value of foods and safeguarding against potential health risks associated with certain cooking methods. While cooking is a fundamental aspect of meal preparation, certain practices can lead to the formation of harmful compounds or the degradation of essential nutrients. Here's a closer look at the importance of steering clear of such practices:

1. Minimizing Overcooking:

Overcooking, particularly at high temperatures, can lead to nutrient degradation. Heat-sensitive vitamins, such as vitamin C and some B vitamins, are vulnerable to breakdown during prolonged or intense cooking. To retain the nutritional value of foods, it's crucial to avoid overcooking vegetables, fruits, and other nutrient-rich ingredients. Opting for gentler cooking methods like steaming, microwaving, or sautéing at lower temperatures helps mitigate nutrient loss.

2. Reducing Charring and Grilling:

Excessive charring or grilling of foods, especially meat, can lead to the formation of potentially harmful compounds, including heterocyclic amines (HCAs) and polycyclic aromatic hydrocarbons (PAHs). These compounds are produced when meat is cooked at high temperatures, such as through grilling or direct flame exposure. Limiting the consumption of heavily charred or grilled foods helps mitigate the potential health risks associated with these compounds, including an increased risk of certain cancers.

3. Moderating the Use of Frying:

While frying can enhance the flavor and texture of foods, excessive use of this cooking method can lead to the formation of harmful trans fats and oxidation of cooking oils.

Trans fats are associated with an increased risk of cardiovascular diseases, and oxidized oils can produce free radicals, contributing to oxidative stress in the body. Moderating the use of frying and choosing healthier cooking oils, such as olive oil or avocado oil, supports both cardiovascular health and overall well-being.

4. Limiting Processed and Packaged Foods:

Processed and packaged foods often undergo cooking methods that involve the use of additives, preservatives, and high levels of sodium. These products may also be exposed to high temperatures during processing, leading to nutrient loss. Opting for fresh, whole foods and minimizing the consumption of heavily processed and packaged items helps reduce the intake of potentially harmful additives and preserves the nutritional quality of the diet.

5. Avoiding Excessive Use of Microwave:

While microwaving is generally considered a safe and efficient cooking method, it's essential to use microwave-safe containers and avoid excessive microwaving, especially in plastic containers that may leach harmful chemicals into food. Using glass or ceramic containers and following recommended guidelines for microwaving ensures the safety of this cooking method.

6. Practicing Food Safety:

Ensuring food safety during cooking is crucial to prevent foodborne illnesses. This includes proper handling, cooking, and storage of perishable foods. Cooking meats to recommended internal temperatures and avoiding cross-contamination are essential practices to reduce the risk of foodborne pathogens.

Avoiding harmful cooking practices is integral to preserving the nutritional quality of foods and minimizing potential health risks associated with certain methods. By adopting mindful cooking techniques and making informed choices in the kitchen, individuals can enjoy meals that are both flavorful and supportive of their overall well-being.

Section 3

Meal Planning for Gut Health

Meal planning is a powerful tool for promoting gut health, as it allows individuals to intentionally choose foods that support digestive well-being and nourish the gut microbiome.

By incorporating a variety of nutrient-dense, fiber-rich, and fermented foods into daily meals, you can create a well-rounded and gut-friendly diet. Here's a closer look at the key aspects of meal planning for gut health:

1. Diverse and Colorful Plate:

Aim for a diverse and colorful plate by incorporating a variety of fruits and vegetables with different colors and textures. These plant-based foods are rich in fiber, vitamins, and antioxidants, promoting overall gut health. Include a mix of leafy greens, cruciferous vegetables, berries, and other colorful produce to provide a wide range of nutrients that support a balanced and thriving gut microbiome.

2. Fiber-Rich Foods:

Prioritize fiber-rich foods in your meal planning as they play a crucial role in supporting digestive health. Whole grains, legumes, nuts, and seeds are excellent sources of dietary fiber. Including a variety of these foods in your meals helps promote regular bowel movements, supports the growth of beneficial gut bacteria, and contributes to a healthy gut environment.

3. Probiotic-Rich Foods:

Incorporate probiotic-rich foods into your meal plan to introduce beneficial bacteria into the gut. Yogurt, kefir, saucrkraut, kimchi, and other fermented foods are excellent sources of probiotics. These foods contribute to a diverse microbiota, enhance digestion, and strengthen the gut's immune function. Including a serving of probiotic-rich foods in your daily meals supports the balance of beneficial bacteria in the gut.

4. Prebiotic Foods:

Don't forget to include prebiotic foods in your meal planning. Prebiotics are non-digestible fibers that nourish the beneficial bacteria in the gut. Foods like garlic, onions, leeks, asparagus, and bananas are rich in prebiotics. By incorporating these foods, you create an environment that promotes the growth and activity of probiotics, fostering a symbiotic relationship for optimal gut health.

5. Balanced Macronutrients:

Ensure a balanced distribution of macronutrients in your meals, including carbohydrates, proteins, and healthy fats. A well-balanced diet provides the necessary building blocks for overall health, including the maintenance of gut tissues and the synthesis of essential compounds. Include sources of lean proteins, whole grains, and healthy fats to create satisfying and nourishing meals.

6. Hydration:

Don't overlook the importance of hydration in gut health. Water is essential for digestion, nutrient absorption, and the overall functioning of the digestive system. Include an adequate amount of water throughout the day and consider incorporating hydrating foods like water-rich fruits and vegetables into your meals.

7. Mindful Eating:

Practice mindful eating as part of your meal planning approach. Paying attention to hunger and fullness cues, savoring the flavors of your food, and avoiding distractions during meals contribute to optimal digestion. Mindful eating can also help reduce stress, which is closely linked to gut health.

By incorporating these principles into your meal planning, you can create a gut-friendly diet that supports digestion, nurtures the gut microbiome, and contributes to overall well-being. Experiment with different recipes, flavors, and food combinations to make your meals both nutritious and enjoyable for optimal gut health.

Weekly Meal Prep Tips

Weekly meal prep is a game-changer for those seeking a convenient, time-efficient, and healthy approach to eating. Planning and preparing meals ahead of time not only saves you from the stress of daily cooking but also ensures that you have nutritious and well-balanced options readily available. Here are some tips to help you master the art of weekly meal prep:

1. Plan Your Menu:

Start by planning your weekly menu. Consider your nutritional needs, dietary preferences, and the number of meals and snacks you'll require.

Choose a variety of recipes to keep your meals interesting, and make sure to include a mix of proteins, carbohydrates, healthy fats, and a rainbow of fruits and vegetables.

2. Create a Shopping List:

Once you've planned your meals, create a detailed shopping list. This list should include all the ingredients you need for your recipes, as well as any staples or snacks you want to have on hand. Organize your list by categories, making your shopping trip more efficient.

3. Invest in Quality Containers:

Having a variety of quality storage containers is crucial for successful meal prep. Choose containers that are both microwave and dishwasher-safe, and opt for different sizes to accommodate various portion sizes. This makes it easy to portion out your meals and store them securely.

4. Batch Cook:

Save time and energy by batch cooking certain components of your meals. For example, cook a large batch of grains, roast a tray of vegetables, or grill several chicken breasts at once. These pre-cooked elements can be mixed and matched throughout the week to create diverse and delicious meals.

5. Use Versatile Ingredients:

Choose versatile ingredients that can be incorporated into multiple meals. For example, roasted sweet potatoes can be added to salads, grain bowls, or wraps. Having a few staple ingredients that work well in different dishes simplifies your meal prep process.

6. Prep in Stages:

Break down your meal prep into manageable stages. For instance, you might dedicate one day to chopping vegetables, another day to cooking proteins, and a third day to assembling and portioning out meals. This makes the process less overwhelming and allows you to tackle different components systematically.

7. Incorporate Freezer-Friendly Options:

Prepare and freeze meals that can be easily reheated when needed. Soups, stews, casseroles, and individually portioned proteins can be stored in the freezer for future use. This provides a convenient option for days when you don't have time to cook.

8. Consider a Theme:

Simplify your weekly meal prep by choosing a theme for the week. For example, you might focus on Mediterranean cuisine one week and Asian-inspired dishes the next. This can streamline your ingredient list and add variety to your meals.

9. Embrace One-Pan Meals:

Opt for one-pan or one-pot meals to minimize cleanup and simplify your cooking process. Sheet pan dinners, casseroles, and stir-fries are excellent options that allow you to combine different ingredients for a complete and fuss-free meal.

10. Stay Flexible:

While planning is essential, stay flexible and be open to making adjustments as needed. Your schedule and preferences may change, so having a degree of flexibility in your meal prep routine allows you to adapt to unforeseen circumstances.

Incorporating these weekly meal prep tips into your routine can save you time, money, and stress while ensuring that you have nourishing and satisfying meals at your fingertips throughout the week.

Creating Balanced and Nutrient-Rich Meals

Creating balanced and nutrient-rich meals is a key component of maintaining overall health and well-being. A well-rounded meal not only satisfies your taste buds but also provides the essential nutrients your body needs for optimal function. Here are some tips to help you craft balanced and nutrient-rich meals:

1. Include a Variety of Food Groups:

Aim to incorporate a variety of food groups into each meal. A balanced plate typically includes a source of lean protein, whole grains, plenty of colorful vegetables, and a serving of healthy fats.

This combination ensures that you get a diverse array of nutrients, including vitamins, minerals, protein, and fiber.

2. Prioritize Colorful Vegetables:

Colorful vegetables are rich in antioxidants, vitamins, and minerals. Different colors often indicate different nutrient profiles, so aim for a mix of vibrant vegetables on your plate. Include a variety of leafy greens, cruciferous vegetables, peppers, carrots, and tomatoes to maximize the nutritional content of your meals.

3. Choose Whole Grains:

Opt for whole grains over refined grains to boost the fiber and nutrient content of your meals. Whole grains like brown rice, quinoa, oats, and whole wheat provide essential carbohydrates, fiber, and various vitamins and minerals. They also contribute to sustained energy levels and promote digestive health.

4. Incorporate Lean Proteins:

Include lean sources of protein in your meals to support muscle health, maintain satiety, and provide essential amino acids. Options like poultry, fish, beans, lentils, tofu, and legumes are excellent choices. Limiting the intake of processed and red meats while diversifying protein sources ensures a well-rounded nutrient profile.

5. Add Healthy Fats:

Incorporate sources of healthy fats, such as avocados, nuts, seeds, and olive oil, to enhance the flavor of your meals and support nutrient absorption. Healthy fats are essential for brain health, hormone production, and overall well-being. Be mindful of portion sizes to maintain balance.

6. Watch Portion Sizes:

Maintain portion control to avoid overeating and to ensure a balanced intake of nutrients. Use smaller plates, listen to your body's hunger and fullness cues, and be mindful of serving sizes to prevent unnecessary calorie consumption.

7. Limit Added Sugars and Processed Foods:

Minimize the consumption of added sugars and highly processed foods, as they often lack essential nutrients and may contribute to health issues when consumed in excess. Choose whole, unprocessed foods to maximize the nutritional value of your meals and support overall health.

8. Hydrate with Water:

Don't forget about hydration. Water is essential for digestion, nutrient absorption, and overall bodily functions. Choose water as your primary beverage and limit the intake of sugary drinks and excessive caffeine.

9. Consider Individual Dietary Needs:

Individual dietary needs vary, so consider any specific dietary requirements or restrictions you may have. Whether you follow a particular eating plan, have allergies, or require modifications, tailor your meals to meet your unique needs while still maintaining balance and nutritional adequacy.

10. Meal Prep for Success:

Plan your meals in advance and engage in meal prep to set yourself up for success. Having nutritious ingredients readily available makes it easier to create balanced meals throughout the week, reducing the temptation to rely on less healthy options.

By following these guidelines and making intentional choices in your meal planning and preparation, you can create meals that are both delicious and packed with the nutrients your body needs for optimal health and vitality.

Section 4

Shopping Guide for Gut Health

Creating a shopping guide for gut health involves making mindful choices to nourish and support your digestive system. The foods you select at the grocery store can have a profound impact on the composition and function of your gut microbiome. Here's a comprehensive shopping guide to help you prioritize gut-friendly options:

1. Fresh Fruits and Vegetables:

Load up your shopping cart with a colorful array of fresh fruits and vegetables. These plant-based foods are rich in fiber, vitamins, and antioxidants that promote gut health. Aim for a variety of options, including leafy greens, berries, apples, cruciferous vegetables, and colorful peppers. These foods not only provide essential nutrients but also serve as prebiotics, nourishing the beneficial bacteria in your gut.

2. Whole Grains:

Choose whole grains over refined grains to boost your fiber intake. Foods like brown rice, quinoa, oats, and whole wheat bread are excellent sources of fiber, which supports regular bowel movements and contributes to a healthy gut environment. Whole grains also provide essential nutrients and energy for your body.

3. Fermented Foods:

Integrate fermented foods into your shopping list to introduce probiotics, beneficial bacteria that support gut health. Yogurt, kefir, sauerkraut, kimchi, and miso are examples of fermented foods that can contribute to a diverse and thriving gut microbiome. Opt for options with live and active cultures for maximum probiotic benefits.

4. Lean Proteins:

Include lean protein sources in your shopping guide for a well-balanced diet. Poultry, fish, tofu, legumes, and beans are excellent choices. Proteins are essential for maintaining and repairing tissues, and incorporating a variety of lean options supports overall digestive health.

5. Nuts and Seeds:

Add nuts and seeds to your shopping list for a dose of healthy fats, fiber, and essential nutrients. Almonds, walnuts, chia seeds, and flaxseeds are particularly beneficial for gut health. These foods contribute to a diverse microbiome and offer additional health benefits, such as anti-inflammatory properties and omega-3 fatty acids.

6. Prebiotic-Rich Foods:

Include prebiotic-rich foods that serve as fuel for beneficial gut bacteria. Garlic, onions, leeks, asparagus, and bananas are excellent choices. These non-digestible fibers promote the growth of probiotics, creating a symbiotic relationship that supports a healthy gut environment.

7. Low-Fat Dairy or Dairy Alternatives:

Choose low-fat dairy products or dairy alternatives fortified with probiotics. These options provide calcium and vitamin D while contributing to a balanced gut microbiome. Be mindful of added sugars in flavored dairy products and opt for plain varieties when possible.

8. Fatty Fish:

Incorporate fatty fish, such as salmon, mackerel, and sardines, into your shopping guide. These fish are rich in omega-3 fatty acids, which have anti-inflammatory properties and support gut health. Omega-3s play a role in maintaining the integrity of the intestinal lining and modulating inflammation in the digestive system.

9. Herbal Teas and Water:

Choose hydrating beverages like water and herbal teas to support digestion. Staying adequately hydrated is essential for overall gut function, aiding in the digestion and absorption of nutrients. Herbal teas, such as peppermint or ginger, can have soothing effects on the digestive system.

10. Limit Processed and Sugary Foods:

Minimize the intake of processed foods and those high in added sugars. These items can negatively impact gut health by promoting the growth of harmful bacteria and contributing to inflammation. Opt for whole, minimally processed foods to provide your gut with the nutrients it needs to thrive.

By incorporating these gut-friendly choices into your shopping routine, you can support a healthy digestive system and foster a diverse and balanced gut microbiome. Remember to focus on variety, freshness, and nutrient density to optimize the impact of your food choices on gut health.

Reading labels is an essential skill when aiming to select gut-friendly products that support digestive health. The information provided on food labels can give insights into the nutritional content, ingredients, and potential impact on the gut microbiome. Here's a guide to help you decipher food labels and make informed choices for a gut-friendly diet:

1. Check the Ingredient List:

Start by examining the ingredient list. Look for whole, minimally processed ingredients, and prioritize foods with recognizable components. Be wary of products with a long list of additives, preservatives, or artificial ingredients, as these may have negative effects on gut health.

2. Look for High Fiber Content:

Fiber is a key component of a gut-friendly diet, supporting regular bowel movements and nourishing beneficial bacteria. Check the label for high fiber content, and choose products that provide a good source of dietary fiber. Whole grains, fruits, vegetables, nuts, and seeds are excellent natural sources of fiber.

3. Probiotic Presence:

Some products, particularly fermented foods and certain dairy items, may contain added probiotics. Check for terms like "live and active cultures" or specific probiotic strains listed in the ingredients. Probiotics contribute to a balanced gut microbiome, promoting the growth of beneficial bacteria.

4. Pay Attention to Sugar Content:

Excessive sugar intake can negatively impact gut health by promoting the growth of harmful bacteria. Check the total sugar content on the label, and be mindful of added sugars and sweeteners. Opt for products with minimal added sugars, especially in items where sweetness may not be necessary.

5. Consider Healthy Fats:

Select products that contain healthy fats, such as monounsaturated and polyunsaturated fats. Look for sources like olive oil, avocados, nuts, and fatty fish. These fats support overall health, including gut health, and contribute to the anti-inflammatory properties of the diet.

6. Be Cautious with Artificial Additives:

Artificial additives, such as artificial colors, flavors, and preservatives, may have adverse effects on the gut. Some individuals may be sensitive to certain additives, which can disrupt the balance of the gut microbiome. Choose products with minimal artificial additives or opt for those with natural alternatives.

7. Mindful Sodium Intake:

High sodium levels can contribute to digestive issues and impact gut health. Check the sodium content on the label, especially in processed and packaged foods. Aim for products with moderate sodium levels and consider incorporating whole, unprocessed foods to help control sodium intake.

8. Identify Allergens:

If you have specific food allergies or intolerances, carefully read labels to identify potential allergens. Common allergens, such as gluten, dairy, nuts, and soy, are often highlighted on food labels. Choosing products that align with your dietary needs helps prevent adverse reactions that may impact gut health.

9. Verify Whole Grain Content:

When selecting grain-based products, ensure they contain whole grains rather than refined grains. Whole grains provide fiber and essential nutrients that contribute to gut health. Look for terms like "whole wheat," "whole oats," or "brown rice" in the ingredient list.

10. Watch for Food Sensitivities:

Be aware of any specific food sensitivities you may have. Reading labels can help you avoid trigger ingredients and make choices that align with your digestive well-being.

Reading labels is a valuable skill for those prioritizing gut health. By focusing on whole, nutrient-dense ingredients, checking for beneficial components like fiber and probiotics, and being mindful of potential additives or allergens, you can make informed choices that contribute to a gut-friendly and nourishing diet.

Choosing Organic and Local Produce

Choosing organic and local produce is a mindful approach to shopping that not only benefits your health but also supports sustainable agriculture and local economies. Organic farming practices prioritize environmental stewardship and avoid synthetic pesticides and fertilizers, while buying local reduces the carbon footprint associated with transportation. Here's why choosing organic and local produce is a positive choice for both individuals and the planet:

1. Organic Produce:

- Reduced Exposure to Pesticides: Organic farming prohibits the use of synthetic pesticides and herbicides. Choosing organic produce reduces your exposure to potentially harmful chemicals commonly used in conventional agriculture. This is particularly important for those seeking to minimize pesticide residues in their diet.

- No Genetically Modified Organisms (GMOs): Organic certification standards typically prohibit the use of genetically modified organisms (GMOs). By choosing organic, you can avoid genetically engineered crops and support agricultural practices that prioritize natural, non-GMO varieties.

- Support for Soil Health: Organic farming practices focus on building and maintaining healthy soil through techniques like crop rotation, cover cropping, and composting. Healthy soil promotes nutrient-rich produce and contributes to the overall sustainability of the agricultural ecosystem.

- Animal Welfare: Organic certification often includes standards for animal welfare. When purchasing organic products, such as dairy or meat, you are supporting farming practices that prioritize the humane treatment of animals, including access to pasture and organic feed.

2. Local Produce:

- ➤ Reduced Carbon Footprint: Buying local produce reduces the distance that food needs to travel from farm to plate. This decreases the carbon footprint associated with transportation and distribution, contributing to lower greenhouse gas emissions. Supporting local farmers also helps to build more resilient and sustainable food systems.

- ➤ Seasonal Variety: Local produce is often harvested at its peak ripeness, providing optimal flavor and nutritional value. By choosing local, you can enjoy a diverse and changing selection of fruits and vegetables that align with the seasons, promoting a varied and nutrient-rich diet.

- ➤ Community Support: Purchasing local produce supports local farmers and strengthens the community economy. This direct connection between consumers and producers fosters a sense of community and enables farmers to receive fair compensation for their products.

- ➤ Preservation of Agricultural Diversity: Supporting local farmers helps preserve agricultural biodiversity. Local farmers often grow a diverse range of crops, contributing to the conservation of different plant varieties and protecting against the potential loss of specific crops due to disease or environmental challenges.

Tips for Choosing Organic and Local Produce:

- ➤ Visit Farmers' Markets: Farmers' markets are excellent places to find local and often organic produce. They provide an opportunity to connect directly with local farmers, ask questions about their farming practices, and discover unique, seasonal offerings.

- ➤ Join a Community Supported Agriculture (CSA) Program: CSA programs allow consumers to subscribe to regular deliveries of fresh, locally grown produce directly from a farm. This model provides support to farmers and offers subscribers a mix of seasonal fruits and vegetables.

- ➤ Check for Organic Certification: Look for the USDA Organic label or other recognized organic certifications when choosing organic produce. These labels indicate that the product meets specific organic standards.

CHAPTER THREE: Gut Friendly Recipes for Women

Section 1

Breakfast Recipes

1. Greek Yogurt Parfait with Berries and Granola:

Ingredients:

1 cup Greek yogurt (preferably unsweetened)

1/2 cup mixed berries (blueberries, strawberries, raspberries)

1/4 cup granola (preferably low-sugar or homemade)

1 tablespoon honey (optional)

Instructions:

In a glass or bowl, layer Greek yogurt, mixed berries, and granola.

Repeat the layers.

Drizzle honey on top if desired.

Enjoy the parfait with a spoon.

Health Benefits:

Greek yogurt provides probiotics for gut health.

Berries are rich in antioxidants and fiber.

Granola adds crunch and additional fiber.

Preparation Time: 5 minutes

2. Avocado Toast with Poached Egg:

Ingredients:

1 slice whole-grain bread

1/2 ripe avocado, mashed

1 poached egg

Salt and pepper to taste

Optional toppings: red pepper flakes, microgreens

Instructions:

Toast the whole-grain bread.

Spread mashed avocado on the toast.

Place the poached egg on top.

Season with salt and pepper.

Add optional toppings as desired.

Health Benefits:

Avocado provides healthy fats.

Whole-grain bread offers fiber.

Poached egg adds protein.

Preparation Time: 10 minutes

3. Berry and Spinach Smoothie Bowl:

Ingredients:

1 cup spinach leaves

1/2 cup mixed berries (strawberries, blueberries)

1/2 banana

1/2 cup Greek yogurt

1/2 cup almond milk

Toppings: chia seeds, sliced almonds, shredded coconut

Instructions:

Blend spinach, berries, banana, Greek yogurt, and almond milk until smooth.

Pour the smoothie into a bowl.

Sprinkle chia seeds, sliced almonds, and shredded coconut on top.

Health Benefits:

Spinach is rich in vitamins and minerals.

Berries offer antioxidants and fiber.

Greek yogurt provides probiotics.

Preparation Time: 5 minutes

4. Quinoa Breakfast Bowl:

Ingredients:

1/2 cup cooked quinoa

1/2 cup mixed berries

1 tablespoon almond butter

1 tablespoon pumpkin seeds

1 teaspoon honey

Instructions:

In a bowl, combine cooked quinoa and mixed berries.

Drizzle almond butter over the mixture.

Sprinkle pumpkin seeds on top.

Drizzle honey for sweetness.

Health Benefits:

Quinoa provides protein and fiber.

Berries offer antioxidants.

Almond butter adds healthy fats.

Preparation Time: 10 minutes

5. Overnight Oats with Almond Milk:

Ingredients:

1/2 cup rolled oats

1/2 cup almond milk

1/2 banana, sliced

1 tablespoon chia seeds

1/4 teaspoon vanilla extract

Instructions:

In a jar, combine rolled oats, almond milk, banana slices, chia seeds, and vanilla extract.

Stir well and refrigerate overnight.

In the morning, give it a good stir and enjoy.

Health Benefits:

Oats provide fiber and prebiotics.

Almond milk is a dairy-free alternative.

Chia seeds offer omega-3 fatty acids.

Preparation Time: 5 minutes (plus overnight soaking)

6. Spinach and Feta Omelette:

Ingredients:

2 eggs

1 cup fresh spinach, chopped

2 tablespoons feta cheese, crumbled

Salt and pepper to taste

1 teaspoon olive oil

Instructions:

In a bowl, whisk eggs and season with salt and pepper.

Heat olive oil in a pan over medium heat.

Add chopped spinach and cook until wilted.

Pour whisked eggs over the spinach.

Sprinkle feta cheese on top.

Cook until the edges set, then fold in half.

Health Benefits:

Spinach is rich in vitamins and iron.

Eggs provide protein.

Feta cheese adds flavor without excessive saturated fat.

Preparation Time: 10 minutes

7. Chia Pudding with Mango:

Ingredients:

2 tablespoons chia seeds

1/2 cup coconut milk

1/2 teaspoon vanilla extract

1/2 cup fresh mango, diced

Instructions:

In a bowl, mix chia seeds, coconut milk, and vanilla extract.

Stir well and refrigerate for at least 2 hours or overnight.

Before serving, top with fresh mango.

Health Benefits:

Chia seeds provide omega-3 fatty acids and fiber.

Coconut milk adds a creamy texture.

Mango offers vitamins and antioxidants.

Preparation Time: 5 minutes (plus chilling time)

8. Sweet Potato and Kale Breakfast Hash:

Ingredients:

1 sweet potato, diced

1 cup kale, chopped

1/4 red onion, diced

2 eggs

1 tablespoon olive oil

Salt and pepper to taste

Instructions:

In a pan, heat olive oil over medium heat.

Add diced sweet potato and cook until tender.

Add chopped kale and red onion, cooking until kale is wilted.

Push the vegetables to the side and crack eggs into the pan.

Cook until eggs reach desired doneness.

Season with salt and pepper and serve.

Health Benefits:

Sweet potatoes provide vitamins and fiber.

Kale is rich in nutrients.

Eggs offer protein and essential amino acids.

Preparation Time: 20 minutes

9. Whole Grain Pancakes with Blueberries:

Ingredients:

1/2 cup whole wheat flour

1/4 cup oats

1/2 teaspoon baking powder

1/2 cup almond milk

1 egg

1/2 cup blueberries

Instructions:

In a bowl, mix whole wheat flour, oats, and baking powder.

Add almond milk and egg, stirring until well combined.

Fold in blueberries.

Heat a griddle or pan and pour batter to make pancakes.

Cook until bubbles form, then flip and cook the other side.

Health Benefits:

Whole wheat flour provides fiber.

Oats offer additional fiber and nutrients.

Blueberries are rich in antioxidants.

Preparation Time: 15 minutes

10. Green Smoothie Bowl:

Ingredients:

1 cup kale or spinach leaves

1/2 banana

1/2 cup pineapple chunks

1/2 cup almond milk

Toppings: sliced kiwi, shredded coconut, chia seeds

Instructions:

Blend kale or spinach, banana, pineapple, and almond milk until smooth.

Pour the smoothie into a bowl.

Top with sliced kiwi, shredded coconut, and chia seeds.

Health Benefits:

Leafy greens provide vitamins and minerals.

Pineapple offers digestive enzymes.

Almond milk adds creaminess without dairy.

Preparation Time: 5 minutes

Section 2

Lunch Recipes

1. Quinoa and Veggie Buddha Bowl

Ingredients:

1 cup cooked quinoa

Mixed vegetables (e.g., broccoli, bell peppers, carrots)

Avocado slices

Chickpeas (canned or cooked)

Tahini dressing

Fresh herbs (parsley or cilantro)

Instructions:

Roast or sauté mixed vegetables until tender.

Assemble the bowl with quinoa, roasted vegetables, avocado slices, and chickpeas.

Drizzle with tahini dressing and sprinkle fresh herbs on top.

Health Benefits:

Quinoa provides protein and fiber.

Mixed vegetables offer vitamins and minerals.

Chickpeas contribute fiber and protein.

Avocado provides healthy fats.

Tahini dressing adds a source of healthy fats.

Preparation Time: 20 minutes

2. Salmon and Avocado Wrap

Ingredients:

Grilled or baked salmon fillet

Whole-grain wrap

Avocado slices

Mixed greens

Greek yogurt sauce (Greek yogurt, lemon juice, dill)

Instructions:

Grill or bake the salmon until cooked.

Lay out the wrap and place salmon, avocado slices, and mixed greens in the center.

Drizzle with Greek yogurt sauce.

Fold the wrap and secure with toothpicks if needed.

Health Benefits:

Salmon provides omega-3 fatty acids.

Avocado offers healthy fats.

Whole-grain wrap adds fiber.

Greek yogurt sauce provides probiotics.

Preparation Time: 15 minutes

3. Chickpea and Spinach Salad

Ingredients:

Canned chickpeas, drained and rinsed

Fresh spinach leaves

Cherry tomatoes, halved

Cucumber, sliced

Feta cheese

Olive oil and balsamic vinegar dressing

Instructions:

In a bowl, combine chickpeas, spinach, cherry tomatoes, cucumber, and feta cheese.

Drizzle with olive oil and balsamic vinegar dressing.

Toss gently to combine.

Health Benefits:

Chickpeas provide fiber and protein.

Spinach offers vitamins and minerals.

Tomatoes contribute antioxidants.

Feta cheese adds calcium.

Preparation Time: 10 minutes

4. Turkey and Quinoa Stuffed Peppers

Ingredients:

Bell peppers, halved and cleaned

Ground turkey

Cooked quinoa

Black beans, drained and rinsed

Diced tomatoes

Taco seasoning

Instructions:

Preheat the oven to 375°F (190°C).

In a skillet, cook ground turkey until browned.

Mix cooked turkey, quinoa, black beans, diced tomatoes, and taco seasoning in a bowl.

Stuff the halved peppers with the mixture.

Bake for 25-30 minutes until peppers are tender.

Health Benefits:

Turkey provides lean protein.

Quinoa adds protein and fiber.

Black beans contribute fiber and antioxidants.

Bell peppers offer vitamins A and C.

Preparation Time: 40 minutes

5. Lentil and Vegetable Stir-Fry

Ingredients:

Cooked lentils

Broccoli florets

Bell peppers, sliced

Snap peas

Carrots, julienned

Soy sauce

Sesame oil

Ginger and garlic, minced

Instructions:

In a wok or skillet, stir-fry broccoli, bell peppers, snap peas, and carrots in sesame oil until crisp-tender.

Add cooked lentils, soy sauce, minced ginger, and garlic.

Stir until well combined and heated through.

Health Benefits:

Lentils provide protein and fiber.

Vegetables offer vitamins and minerals.

Soy sauce adds flavor without excess salt.

Preparation Time: 25 minutes

Ingredients:

Cooked quinoa

Cucumber, diced

Cherry tomatoes, halved

Kalamata olives, sliced

Feta cheese

Red onion, finely chopped

Greek dressing (olive oil, lemon juice, oregano)

Instructions:

In a bowl, combine quinoa, cucumber, cherry tomatoes, olives, feta cheese, and red onion.

Drizzle with Greek dressing and toss gently to combine.

Health Benefits:

Quinoa provides protein and fiber.

Cucumber and tomatoes offer hydration and vitamins.

Olives add healthy fats.

Feta cheese provides calcium.

Preparation Time: 15 minutes

7. Sweet Potato and Chickpea Bowl

Ingredients:

Roasted sweet potatoes, cubed

Canned chickpeas, drained and rinsed

Spinach leaves

Cherry tomatoes, halved

Avocado slices

Lemon-tahini dressing

Instructions:

Roast sweet potatoes and chickpeas until golden.

Assemble a bowl with spinach, roasted sweet potatoes, chickpeas, cherry tomatoes, and avocado slices.

Drizzle with lemon-tahini dressing.

Health Benefits:

Sweet potatoes provide vitamins and fiber.

Chickpeas offer protein and fiber.

Spinach adds iron and other nutrients.

Avocado contributes healthy fats.

Preparation Time: 30 minutes

8. Shrimp and Quinoa Stir-Fry

Ingredients:

Shrimp, peeled and deveined

Cooked quinoa

Broccoli florets

Bell peppers, sliced

Snow peas

Low-sodium soy sauce

Garlic and ginger, minced

Instructions:

In a wok or skillet, stir-fry shrimp, broccoli, bell peppers, and snow peas until shrimp is cooked.

Add cooked quinoa, soy sauce, minced garlic, and ginger.

Stir until well combined and heated through.

Health Benefits:

Shrimp provides a lean source of protein.

Quinoa adds protein and fiber.

Vegetables offer vitamins and minerals.

Soy sauce adds flavor without excess sodium.

Preparation Time: 20 minutes

9. Mediterranean Hummus Wrap

Ingredients:

Whole-grain wrap

Hummus

Grilled chicken strips

Cherry tomatoes, halved

Cucumber, sliced

Red onion, thinly sliced

Fresh parsley, chopped

Instructions:

Spread hummus on the whole-grain wrap.

Layer with grilled chicken strips, cherry tomatoes, cucumber, red onion, and fresh parsley.

Roll up the wrap and secure with toothpicks if needed.

Health Benefits:

Whole-grain wrap provides fiber.

Hummus offers plant-based protein.

Grilled chicken adds lean protein.

Vegetables contribute vitamins and minerals.

Preparation Time: 15 minutes

10. Vegetable and Tofu Stir-Fry

Ingredients:

Firm tofu, cubed

Broccoli florets

Carrots, julienned

Snap peas

Red bell pepper, sliced

Low-sodium soy sauce

Sesame oil

Garlic and ginger, minced

Instructions:

In a wok or skillet, stir-fry tofu, broccoli, carrots, snap peas, and bell pepper in sesame oil until tofu is golden.

Add minced garlic, ginger, and soy sauce.

Stir until well combined and heated through.

Health Benefits:

Tofu provides plant-based protein.

Vegetables offer vitamins and minerals.

Soy sauce adds flavor without excess salt.

Preparation Time: 25 minutes

Section 3

Dinner Recipes

1. Grilled Salmon with Quinoa and Roasted Vegetables:

Ingredients:

Salmon fillets

Quinoa

Assorted vegetables (bell peppers, zucchini, cherry tomatoes)

Olive oil

Lemon

Garlic

Fresh herbs (thyme, rosemary)

Instructions:

Preheat the grill and oven.

Marinate salmon with olive oil, lemon juice, minced garlic, and herbs.

Grill salmon until cooked through.

Roast vegetables in the oven with olive oil and herbs.

Cook quinoa according to package instructions.

Serve grilled salmon over a bed of quinoa and roasted vegetables.

Health Benefits:

Salmon is rich in omega-3 fatty acids for heart health.

Quinoa provides fiber and essential amino acids.

Colorful vegetables offer a variety of antioxidants.

Preparation Time: Approximately 30 minutes.

2. Chickpea and Spinach Curry:

Ingredients:

Chickpeas (canned or cooked)

Spinach

Onion

Garlic

Ginger

Tomatoes

Coconut milk

Curry spices (turmeric, cumin, coriander, garam masala)

Basmati rice

Instructions:

Sauté onions, garlic, and ginger in a pan.

Add curry spices and cook until fragrant.

Stir in chickpeas, diced tomatoes, and coconut milk.

Simmer until the curry thickens.

Add fresh spinach and cook until wilted.

Serve over cooked basmati rice.

Health Benefits:

Chickpeas provide plant-based protein and fiber.

Spinach is rich in iron and vitamins.

Turmeric and ginger have anti-inflammatory properties.

Preparation Time: Approximately 40 minutes.

3. Quinoa Salad with Mixed Greens and Avocado:

Ingredients:

Quinoa

Mixed salad greens (spinach, arugula, kale)

Cherry tomatoes

Cucumber

Avocado

Feta cheese

Olive oil

Balsamic vinegar

Dijon mustard

Instructions:

Cook quinoa according to package instructions.

Chop vegetables and avocado.

In a bowl, mix cooked quinoa, vegetables, avocado, and feta.

Whisk together olive oil, balsamic vinegar, and Dijon mustard for the dressing.

Drizzle dressing over the salad and toss gently.

Health Benefits:

Quinoa offers protein and fiber.

Leafy greens provide vitamins and minerals.

Avocado contributes healthy fats.

Preparation Time: Approximately 25 minutes.

4. Turkey and Vegetable Stir-Fry:

Ingredients:

Ground turkey

Broccoli

Bell peppers (various colors)

Snow peas

Carrots

Garlic

Soy sauce

Sesame oil

Brown rice

Instructions:

In a wok or skillet, brown ground turkey.

Add minced garlic and stir.

Add chopped vegetables and stir-fry until crisp-tender.

Pour in soy sauce and sesame oil, toss to coat.

Serve over cooked brown rice.

Health Benefits:

Lean turkey provides protein.

Colorful vegetables offer vitamins and antioxidants.

Brown rice provides fiber and complex carbohydrates.

Preparation Time: Approximately 30 minutes.

Ingredients:

Lentils

Onion

Carrots

Celery

Garlic

Vegetable broth

Tomatoes

Spinach

Thyme

Bay leaves

Instructions:

Sauté onions, garlic, carrots, and celery in a pot.

Add lentils, tomatoes, thyme, and bay leaves.

Pour in vegetable broth and bring to a boil.

Simmer until lentils are tender.

Stir in fresh spinach before serving.

Health Benefits:

Lentils are a good source of protein and fiber.

Vegetables provide vitamins and minerals.

Spinach adds iron and antioxidants.

Preparation Time: Approximately 45 minutes.

6. Baked Cod with Lemon and Herbs:

Ingredients:

Cod fillets

Lemon

Fresh herbs (parsley, dill)

Garlic

Olive oil

Cherry tomatoes

Asparagus

Instructions:

Preheat the oven.

Place cod fillets on a baking sheet.

Drizzle with olive oil and lemon juice.

Sprinkle with minced garlic and fresh herbs.

Arrange cherry tomatoes and asparagus around the cod.

Bake until the fish is flaky.

Health Benefits:

Cod is a lean source of protein.

Asparagus provides fiber and folate.

Lemon and herbs add flavor without extra calories.

Preparation Time: Approximately 20 minutes.

Ingredients:

Sweet potatoes

Black beans

Onion

Garlic

Cumin, chili powder, paprika

Whole wheat tortillas

Enchilada sauce

Cheese (optional)

Instructions:

Roast sweet potatoes and black beans with spices.

Sauté onions and garlic until soft.

Mix sweet potato mixture with sautéed onions.

Spoon the mixture into whole wheat tortillas.

Roll and place in a baking dish, top with enchilada sauce.

Optionally, sprinkle with cheese.

Bake until bubbly and golden.

Health Benefits:

Sweet potatoes are rich in vitamins and fiber.

Black beans provide protein and fiber.

Whole wheat tortillas offer complex carbohydrates.

Preparation Time: Approximately 45 minutes.

8. Mediterranean Quinoa Bowl:

Ingredients:

Quinoa

Chickpeas

Cucumber

Cherry tomatoes

Red onion

Kalamata olives

Feta cheese

Olive oil

Lemon juice

Fresh oregano

Instructions:

Cook quinoa according to package instructions.

Assemble bowls with quinoa, chickpeas, chopped vegetables, olives, and feta.

Drizzle with olive oil and lemon juice.

Sprinkle with fresh oregano.

Health Benefits:

Quinoa provides protein and fiber.

Chickpeas offer plant-based protein.

Mediterranean ingredients provide healthy fats and antioxidants.

Preparation Time: Approximately 25 minutes.

9. Shrimp and Vegetable Skewers:

Ingredients:

Shrimp (peeled and deveined)

Bell peppers (various colors)

Red onion

Zucchini

Cherry tomatoes

Olive oil

Garlic

Lemon

Fresh herbs (parsley, thyme)

Instructions:

Preheat the grill.

Thread shrimp and chopped vegetables onto skewers.

Mix olive oil, minced garlic, lemon juice, and herbs for a marinade.

Brush the skewers with the marinade.

Grill until shrimp are cooked through.

Health Benefits:

Shrimp is a low-calorie source of protein.

Colorful vegetables offer vitamins and antioxidants.

Olive oil provides heart healthy monounsaturated fats.

Preparation Time: Approximately 20 minutes.

Ingredients:

Arborio rice

Butternut squash

Kale

Onion

Garlic

Vegetable broth

White wine

Parmesan cheese

Olive oil

Instructions:

Sauté onions and garlic in olive oil.

Add Arborio rice and stir until coated.

Pour in white wine and cook until absorbed.

Gradually add vegetable broth, stirring constantly.

Stir in diced butternut squash and chopped kale.

Continue cooking until rice is creamy.

Finish with grated Parmesan cheese.

Health Benefits:

Butternut squash is rich in vitamins A and C.

Kale provides fiber, vitamins, and minerals.

Arborio rice offers complex carbohydrates.

Preparation Time: Approximately 40 minutes.

Section 4

Snack Recipes

1. Greek Yogurt Parfait:

Ingredients:

1 cup Greek yogurt (unsweetened)

1/2 cup mixed berries (blueberries, strawberries, raspberries)

2 tablespoons granola

1 tablespoon honey

Instructions:

In a glass or bowl, layer Greek yogurt.

Add a layer of mixed berries.

Sprinkle granola on top.

Drizzle honey over the parfait.

Repeat the layers if desired.

Health Benefits:

Greek yogurt provides probiotics for gut health.

Berries are rich in antioxidants and fiber.

Granola adds fiber and crunch.

Preparation TIme: 5 minutes

2. Avocado and Whole Grain Crackers:

Ingredients:

1 ripe avocado

Whole grain crackers

Instructions:

Mash the avocado in a bowl.

Spread mashed avocado on whole grain crackers.

Health Benefits:

Avocado is a source of healthy fats.

Whole grain crackers provide fiber.

Preparation Time: 3 minutes

3. Roasted Chickpeas:

Ingredients:

1 can chickpeas (drained and rinsed)

1 tablespoon olive oil

1 teaspoon paprika

1/2 teaspoon cumin

Salt to taste

Instructions:

Preheat oven to 400°F (200°C).

In a bowl, toss chickpeas with olive oil, paprika, cumin, and salt.

Spread chickpeas on a baking sheet.

Roast for 20-25 minutes until crispy.

Health Benefits:

Chickpeas are a good source of fiber and protein.

Preparation Time: 30 minutes

4. Green Smoothie:

Ingredients:

1 cup spinach

1/2 banana

1/2 cup pineapple chunks

1/2 cup Greek yogurt

1/2 cup water or coconut water

Instructions:

Blend all ingredients until smooth.

Health Benefits:

Spinach provides fiber and vitamins.

Greek yogurt adds probiotics.

Pineapple offers digestive enzymes.

Preparation Time: 5 minutes

5. Homemade Trail Mix:

Ingredients:

Almonds

Walnuts

Pumpkin seeds

Dried cranberries

Dark chocolate chips

Instructions:

Mix all ingredients in a bowl.

Portion into snack-sized bags.

Health Benefits:

Nuts and seeds provide healthy fats and fiber.

Dark chocolate offers antioxidants.

Preparation Time: 5 minutes

6. Cucumber Slices with Hummus:

Ingredients:

Cucumber, sliced

Hummus

Instructions:

Slice cucumber into rounds.

Dip cucumber slices into hummus.

Health Benefits:

Cucumbers are hydrating and low-calorie.

Hummus provides fiber and protein.

Preparation Time: 5 minutes

7. Chia Seed Pudding:

Ingredients:

2 tablespoons chia seeds

1/2 cup almond milk

1/2 teaspoon vanilla extract

Fresh berries for topping

Instructions:

Mix chia seeds, almond milk, and vanilla extract in a jar.

Refrigerate for at least 2 hours or overnight.

Top with fresh berries before serving.

Health Benefits:

Chia seeds are rich in fiber and omega-3 fatty acids.

Preparation Time: 2 hours (including chilling time)

8. Kale Chips:

Ingredients:

Fresh kale, washed and dried

Olive oil

Sea salt

Instructions:

Preheat oven to 275°F (135°C).

Tear kale into bite-sized pieces.

Toss with olive oil and sprinkle with sea salt.

Bake for 20-25 minutes until crispy.

Health Benefits:

Kale is a nutrient-dense leafy green.

Preparation Time: 30 minutes

9. Apple Slices with Almond Butter:

Ingredients:

Apple, sliced

Almond butter

Instructions:

Spread almond butter on apple slices.

Health Benefits:

Apples provide fiber and antioxidants.

Almond butter adds healthy fats and protein.

Preparation Time: 5 minutes

10. Turmeric Yogurt Dip with Veggie Sticks:

Ingredients:

1 cup Greek yogurt

1 teaspoon turmeric powder

1/2 teaspoon cumin

Assorted vegetable sticks (carrots, bell peppers, celery)

Instructions:

Mix Greek yogurt, turmeric, and cumin in a bowl.

Use as a dip for vegetable sticks.

Health Benefits:

Turmeric has anti-inflammatory properties.

Greek yogurt provides probiotics.

Preparation Time: 5 minutes

Ingredients:

2 pounds of grass-fed beef or organic chicken bones

2 carrots, chopped

2 celery stalks, chopped

1 onion, peeled and halved

4 cloves of garlic, minced

2 tablespoons apple cider vinegar

Fresh herbs (rosemary, thyme)

Salt and pepper to taste

Instructions:

Place bones in a large pot and cover with water.

Add vegetables, garlic, apple cider vinegar, and herbs.

Bring to a boil, then simmer for at least 8 hours.

Strain and season with salt and pepper.

Health Benefits:

Bone broth is rich in collagen, amino acids, and minerals, supporting gut health and reducing inflammation.

Preparation Time: 10 minutes (prep), 8 hours (cooking)

2. Gut-Healing Miso Soup:

Ingredients:

4 cups vegetable broth

2 tablespoons miso paste

1 cup sliced shiitake mushrooms

1 cup baby spinach

1 tablespoon grated ginger

2 green onions, chopped

1 block tofu, cubed

Instructions:

Heat broth in a pot, but do not boil.

In a bowl, mix miso paste with a bit of warm broth until smooth.

Add miso mixture, mushrooms, tofu, ginger, and spinach to the pot.

Simmer until vegetables are tender.

Garnish with green onions.

Health Benefits:

Miso is a fermented food that provides probiotics, supporting gut microbiota.

Preparation Time: 20 minutes

3. Turmeric and Ginger Lentil Stew:

Ingredients:

1 cup lentils, rinsed

4 cups vegetable broth

1 onion, chopped

2 carrots, diced

2 celery stalks, chopped

3 cloves garlic, minced

1 tablespoon turmeric

1 tablespoon grated ginger

1 teaspoon cumin

Salt and pepper to taste

Instructions:

In a pot, combine lentils, broth, vegetables, and spices.

Bring to a boil, then simmer until lentils are tender.

Adjust seasonings and serve.

Health Benefits:

Turmeric and ginger have anti-inflammatory properties, promoting gut health.

Preparation Time: 30 minutes

4. Coconut Milk and Veggie Curry Soup:

Ingredients:

1 can coconut milk

4 cups vegetable broth

1 sweet potato, diced

1 zucchini, sliced

1 red bell pepper, chopped

1 cup snap peas

2 tablespoons red curry paste

1 tablespoon coconut oil

Fresh cilantro for garnish

Instructions:

In a pot, sauté vegetables in coconut oil.

Add coconut milk, broth, and curry paste.

Simmer until vegetables are cooked.

Garnish with cilantro before serving.

Health Benefits:

Coconut milk provides healthy fats, and the vegetables offer fiber for gut health.

Preparation Time: 25 minutes

5. Quinoa and Vegetable Stew:

Ingredients:

1 cup quinoa, rinsed

4 cups vegetable broth

1 onion, chopped

2 carrots, sliced

2 cups broccoli florets

1 can diced tomatoes

2 cloves garlic, minced

1 teaspoon dried oregano

Salt and pepper to taste

Instructions:

Combine quinoa, broth, vegetables, tomatoes, and spices in a pot.

Bring to a boil, then simmer until quinoa is cooked.

Season to taste and serve.

Health Benefits:

Quinoa is a good source of fiber and protein, supporting gut health and satiety.

Preparation Time: 30 minutes

6. Gut-Friendly Chickpea and Spinach Stew:

Ingredients:

2 cans chickpeas, drained

4 cups vegetable broth

1 onion, chopped

3 tomatoes, diced

4 cups baby spinach

3 cloves garlic, minced

1 teaspoon cumin

1 teaspoon paprika

Olive oil for sautéing

Instructions:

Sauté onions and garlic in olive oil until softened.

Add tomatoes, chickpeas, broth, and spices.

Simmer until flavors meld.

Stir in spinach until wilted.

Health Benefits:

Chickpeas provide fiber, and spinach is rich in vitamins, promoting gut health.

Preparation Time: 25 minutes

7. Gut-Nourishing Chicken and Vegetable Soup:

Ingredients:

2 chicken breasts, cooked and shredded

6 cups chicken broth

2 carrots, sliced

2 celery stalks, chopped

1 onion, diced

2 cloves garlic, minced

1 cup green beans, chopped

Fresh dill for garnish

Salt and pepper to taste

Instructions:

In a pot, sauté onions and garlic until fragrant.

Add chicken, broth, vegetables, and seasonings.

Simmer until vegetables are tender.

Garnish with fresh dill before serving.

Health Benefits:

Chicken provides lean protein, and the vegetables offer a variety of vitamins and minerals.

Preparation Time: 40 minutes

Ingredients:

4 leeks, sliced

3 potatoes, peeled and diced

4 cups vegetable broth

1 cup almond milk

2 tablespoons olive oil

1 teaspoon thyme

Salt and pepper to taste

Instructions:

Sauté leeks in olive oil until softened.

Add potatoes, broth, almond milk, and thyme.

Simmer until potatoes are tender.

Blend until smooth and season to taste.

Health Benefits:

Potatoes provide resistant starch, and leeks offer prebiotics for gut health.

Preparation Time: 35 minutes

9. Cabbage and Turmeric Detox Soup:

Ingredients:

1 small head of cabbage, shredded

1 onion, chopped

3 carrots, sliced

4 cups vegetable broth

1 tablespoon turmeric

1 tablespoon apple cider vinegar

Fresh parsley for garnish

Salt and pepper to taste

Instructions:

Sauté onions in olive oil until translucent.

Add cabbage, carrots, broth, turmeric, and apple cider vinegar.

Simmer until vegetables are tender.

Garnish with fresh parsley before serving.

Health Benefits:

Cabbage supports detoxification, and turmeric has anti-inflammatory properties.

Preparation Time: 30 minutes

10. Gut-Healing Lentil and Kale Stew:

Ingredients:

1 cup green or brown lentils, rinsed

1 bunch kale, stems removed and chopped

4 cups vegetable broth

1 onion, diced

2 carrots, diced

2 cloves garlic, minced

1 teaspoon cumin

1 teaspoon smoked paprika

Olive oil for sautéing

Lemon wedges for serving

Instructions:

Sauté onions and garlic in olive oil until softened.

Add lentils, broth, vegetables, and spices.

Simmer until lentils are cooked and kale is tender.

Serve with a squeeze of lemon.

Health Benefits:

Lentils provide fiber, and kale is rich in vitamins and minerals, supporting gut health.

Preparation Time: 35 minutes

Fermented Beverages Recipes

1. Kombucha:

Ingredients:

4 black tea bags

1 cup of white sugar

SCOBY (Symbiotic Culture of Bacteria and Yeast)

1 cup of starter tea (previously brewed kombucha)

Instructions:

Brew the black tea and dissolve sugar in hot tea.

Allow the tea to cool, remove the tea bags, and transfer to a large jar.

Add the SCOBY and starter tea.

Cover with a cloth and secure with a rubber band.

Ferment for 7-21 days, depending on taste preference.

Bottle and refrigerate.

Health Benefits:

Kombucha is rich in probiotics, aiding digestion and promoting a healthy gut microbiome.

Preparation Time: 20-30 minutes (plus fermentation time).

2. Ginger Water Kefir:

Ingredients:

Water kefir grains

4 cups of water

1/4 cup of organic cane sugar

1-inch piece of fresh ginger, grated

Instructions:

Dissolve sugar in water and cool to room temperature.

Add water kefir grains and grated ginger to a glass jar.

Pour in the sugar water.

Cover and ferment for 24-48 hours.

Strain and transfer liquid to a bottle.

Refrigerate before serving.

Health Benefits:

Water kefir is a probiotic beverage that supports gut health, while ginger provides anti-inflammatory properties.

Preparation Time: 10-15 minutes (plus fermentation time).

3. Fermented Beet Kvass:

Ingredients:

2-3 medium beets, peeled and chopped

1 tablespoon sea salt

Filtered water

Instructions:

Place beets in a glass jar.

Dissolve salt in water and pour over the beets.

Cover the jar and ferment for 5-7 days.

Strain and transfer liquid to a bottle.

Refrigerate before serving.

Health Benefits:

Beet kvass is rich in probiotics, supports liver function, and provides essential nutrients.

Preparation Time: 15-20 minutes (plus fermentation time).

4. Blueberry Jun Tea:

Ingredients:

4 green tea bags

1 cup honey

SCOBY

1 cup starter tea

1 cup fresh blueberries

Instructions:

Brew the green tea and dissolve honey in hot tea.

Allow the tea to cool, remove the tea bags, and transfer to a large jar.

Add the SCOBY and starter tea.

Add fresh blueberries.

Cover with a cloth and secure with a rubber band.

Ferment for 7-21 days.

Bottle and refrigerate.

Health Benefits:

Blueberries are rich in antioxidants, while jun tea provides probiotics and enzymes.

Preparation Time: 20-30 minutes (plus fermentation time).

5. Pineapple Ginger Water Kefir:

Ingredients:

Water kefir grains

4 cups of coconut water

1/4 cup of organic cane sugar

1 cup fresh pineapple, diced

1-inch piece of fresh ginger, sliced

Instructions:

Dissolve sugar in coconut water and cool to room temperature.

Add water kefir grains to a glass jar.

Pour in the sugar water.

Add diced pineapple and sliced ginger.

Cover and ferment for 24-48 hours.

Strain and transfer liquid to a bottle.

Refrigerate before serving.

Health Benefits:

Coconut water provides electrolytes, while pineapple and ginger offer digestive benefits.

Preparation Time: 15-20 minutes (plus fermentation time).

6. Cranberry Orange Kombucha:

Ingredients:

4 black tea bags

1 cup of white sugar

SCOBY

1 cup starter tea

1 cup fresh cranberries

Zest of one orange

Instructions:

Brew the black tea and dissolve sugar in hot tea.

Allow the tea to cool, remove the tea bags, and transfer to a large jar.

Add the SCOBY and starter tea.

Add fresh cranberries and orange zest.

Cover with a cloth and secure with a rubber band.

Ferment for 7-21 days.

Bottle and refrigerate.

Health Benefits:

Cranberries are known for their anti-inflammatory properties, and the orange provides vitamin C.

Preparation Time: 20-30 minutes (plus fermentation time).

7. Hibiscus Ginger Water Kefir:

Ingredients:

Water kefir grains

4 cups of water

1/4 cup of organic cane sugar

2 tablespoons dried hibiscus flowers

1-inch piece of fresh ginger, grated

Instructions:

Dissolve sugar in water and cool to room temperature.

Add water kefir grains to a glass jar.

Pour in the sugar water.

Add dried hibiscus flowers and grated ginger.

Cover and ferment for 24-48 hours.

Strain and transfer liquid to a bottle.

Refrigerate before serving.

Health Benefits:

Hibiscus is rich in antioxidants, and ginger provides anti-inflammatory and digestive benefits.

Preparation Time: 15-20 minutes (plus fermentation time).

8. Mint Lemonade Kombucha:

Ingredients:

4 green tea bags

1 cup of white sugar

SCOBY

1 cup starter tea

1 cup fresh mint leaves

Juice of 2 lemons

Instructions:

Brew the green tea and dissolve sugar in hot tea.

Allow the tea to cool, remove the tea bags, and transfer to a large jar.

Add the SCOBY and starter tea.

Add fresh mint leaves and lemon juice.

Cover with a cloth and secure with a rubber band.

Ferment for 7-21 days.

Bottle and refrigerate.

Health Benefits:

Mint aids digestion, while lemon provides vitamin C and adds a refreshing flavor.

Preparation Time: 20-30 minutes (plus fermentation time).

9. Mango Turmeric Water Kefir:

Ingredients:

Water kefir grains

4 cups of coconut water

1/4 cup of organic cane sugar

1 cup fresh mango, diced

1-inch piece of fresh turmeric, grated

Instructions:

Dissolve sugar in coconut water and cool to room temperature.

Add water kefir grains to a glass jar.

Pour in the sugar water.

Add diced mango and grated turmeric.

Cover and ferment for 24-48 hours.

Strain and transfer liquid to a bottle.

Refrigerate before serving.

Health Benefits:

Mango provides natural sweetness, while turmeric offers anti-inflammatory properties.

Preparation Time: 15-20 minutes (plus fermentation time).

10. Raspberry Rose Jun Tea:

Ingredients:

4 green tea bags

1 cup honey

SCOBY

1 cup starter tea

1 cup fresh raspberries

1 tablespoon dried rose petals

Instructions:

Brew the green tea and dissolve honey in hot tea.

Allow the tea to cool, remove the tea bags, and transfer to a large jar.

Add the SCOBY and starter tea.

Add fresh raspberries and dried rose petals.

Cover with a cloth and secure with a rubber band.

Ferment for 7-21 days.

Bottle and refrigerate.

Health Benefits:

Raspberries are rich in antioxidants, and rose petals add a delicate flavor.

Preparation Time: 20-30 minutes (plus fermentation time).

CONCLUSION

This Gut Health Cookbook for Women serves as a comprehensive guide to nourishing both body and mind through mindful and delicious culinary choices. By embracing the principles of gut-friendly nutrition, you embark on a journey to cultivate a thriving microbiome, enhance digestion, and promote overall well-being.

Throughout these pages, we've explored a diverse array of recipes featuring gut-loving ingredients – from fiber-rich foods and fermented delights to prebiotic-rich plant-based dishes. These recipes are not just meals; they are invitations to prioritize your health, finding joy in the vibrant colors, flavors, and textures that contribute to a balanced and nourishing diet.

Understanding the importance of cooking techniques, choosing organic and local produce, and deciphering food labels empowers you to make informed decisions that align with your wellness goals. The recipes provided not only tantalize the taste buds but also offer a symphony of nutrients that support your gut, your body's intricate ecosystem.

As you embark on this culinary adventure, remember that achieving and maintaining gut health is a holistic journey. It involves a harmonious blend of nutrition, mindfulness, and self-care. Listen to your body's cues, savor the moments spent in the kitchen, and relish the satisfaction of creating meals that contribute to your overall vitality.

May this cookbook inspire you to explore the world of gut-friendly cuisine, sparking creativity in your kitchen and fostering a deeper connection with the foods you consume. The journey to gut health is a personal and ongoing one, and with these recipes, tips, and insights, you're equipped with the tools to make every meal a nourishing and delightful experience.

Here's to a future filled with vibrant health, gastronomic pleasure, and the joy that comes from knowing you are actively contributing to the well-being of your gut and, consequently, your entire being. Happy cooking, happy eating, and may your gut flourish with the abundance of goodness you've cultivated within these pages. Cheers to a life of wellness and delicious exploration!